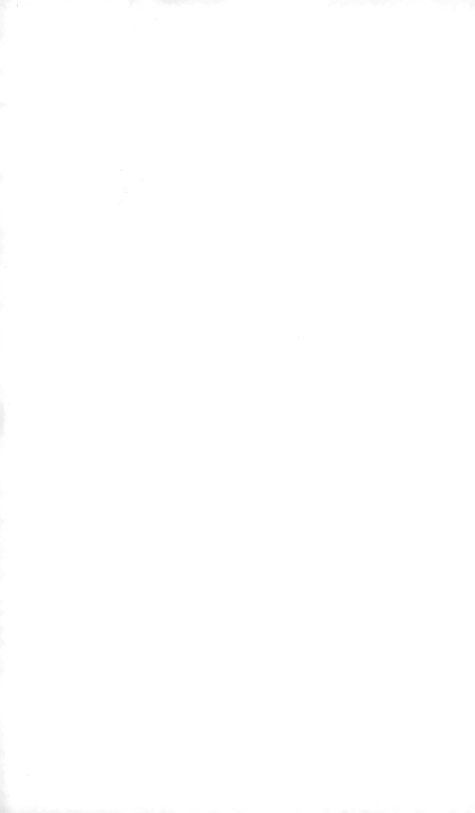

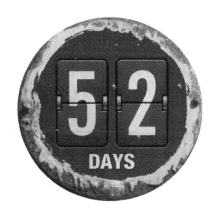

Countdown to Your Best Body
Success Journal

Sohailla Digsby, RD, LD

Book design by
Daniel R. Pearson
dan@augustarx.com

ISBN-13: 978-1494878979
ISBN-10: 1494878976

Printed in the United States of America

The information in this book, while believed to be true and accurate, is presented for informational purposes only and is not intended to diagnose or treat any medical condition. For specific medical advice, diagnosis and treatment, consult your doctor or other healthcare professional.

Contents

Let the Countdown begin!

As you work through this Success Journal, you will soon find yourself in a place where your body does not hold you back from being your very best. How do you know if your body is holding you back from living life to the fullest? If you aren't comfortable in your own skin (or last year's wardrobe), if you feel out of control when it comes to food, if you can't move quickly without huffing and puffing, or if you are heading down the path of increasing medications, doctor's visits, and bills, then you are being held back! Perhaps you have been at your personal best before, but it was much too brief for your satisfaction. Or perhaps it was so long ago that you can only remember it because it was on your wedding day.

I am excited to begin this journey with you - leading you to Your Best Body! After 15 years of working with nutrition clients and fitness class participants, many of whom struggle with their weight and with consistency, I have compiled what, in my experience, has proven to bring the greatest success. Be assured that the Countdown in this Success Journal will set you up for reaching Your Best Body, and staying there for good. Imagine always being at your BEST, both inside and out! This tool will help you build a lifetime of healthy habits one realistic yet challenging step at a time, while seeing and feeling results along the way.

To reach Your Best Body, plan to give the challenges assigned to each day your very best effort for 52 days straight! Why 52 days?

Psychologists say that it takes about a month to set up new habits. However, most people need a little longer than that to see the kind of "Best Body" results they are after...52 days is about 2 months.

Although I am not a psychologist, I am a registered dietitian/ nutritionist, a fitness instructor, and a "chef" to an active household. For many years I have listened closely to the stories and struggles of many who have the same goal as you: to reach their Best Body.

I see the confusion that is in the marketplace related to nutrition and exercise, and hear how frustrating it is for my clients. There are many promises for quick fixes made by those perhaps only looking at dollar signs and not considering how their recommendations will affect your overall health and future weight maintenance efforts. Some give advice from pamphlets and testimonials that they have read, but hopefully their mispronunciation of the basic terms of nutrition science flags you to bypass their advice relating to your personal health. There are many giving nutrition advice who know the research, but do not interact with those to whom they are penning their recommendations, so they don't foresee the pitfalls. There are also those who actually consult with the health-seekers; however, they do not have any personal experience doing the work of getting and staying fit. You can be assured that "I get it" because every day, I am fleshing out the very challenges you are about to take on. I know it is not always easy to stay committed for 52 days, but as you will find, it is most certainly worthwhile.

My approach is both research-based and experience-based. My recommendations take the facts from the current literature, as well as feedback from people just like you, providing you with practical tools that really work. One of my favorite aspects of nutrition counseling is investigating what exactly is responsible for the shortfall of ongoing success in each unique person. The Countdown challenges I have chosen share my secrets to success! They unveil the blueprints that my clients, who I see all around town sporting their Best Bodies year after year, now live by. The challenges, and the order in which they are presented to you through this Countdown, are intended to alert you to what no other diet, book, or program has personally explored with you.

Many of my clients were "doing things right" when they started, but without the results they desired. However, they have been able to identify through the daily Countdown challenges and the journaling of this program just what has been holding them back from reaching their very Best Bodies. I have found that most people who have completed this program can quickly identify one or two days' specific challenges that were game-changers for them...ones they would have never discovered without doing all 52 days of the Best Body Countdown.

This approach will help you to build section upon section of the fortress that protects your health, keeping in mind what the finished masterpiece will be like when it is complete. Plan to see the Countdown through until you have reached Your Best Body. Understand that those with a lot of weight to lose will not reach their final Best Body destination in just 52 days. In that case, plan to repeat the 52 day Countdown until you have reached your goal. It gets easier!

Ultimately, your success depends on you. Those who have completed this program and have a Success Journal full of check-marks for each day's challenges, also have a pantry that looks as different from 52 days ago as they do in their jeans (both look AMAZING post-Countdown). Taking small steps to make a few daily changes will bring you long-term results. Real change is not instant, but with this approach, it is lasting.

For most readers, reaching your Best Body destination requires weight loss. Weight lost during this Countdown will not be water weight or muscle weight - just the fluffy, jiggly, over-your-waistband kind of stuff that you want gone. It would be wrong of me to encourage weight loss strategies that have you reaching Your Best Body goal weight by way of dehydration, diarrhea, and muscle atrophy. I know that you want the numbers to drop fast, but I don't want my 52 day Countdown winners to be dehydrated, mushy-muscle "losers."

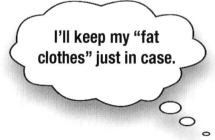

I'll keep my "fat clothes" just in case.

I can hear some of you thinking this. Don't do it! Keep two sizes in succession so you can stay in a reasonable 3-5 pound range. Seriously. This is it.

9

If you could see what I have seen over many years of working in the weight loss and wellness industry, you would most definitely choose the ideal weekly 1 to 3 pounds of fat tissue loss instead of greater weekly loss (most of which is water and muscle loss). You would be convinced that it just doesn't last. Unfortunately, however, often what is lasting is your compromised metabolism, making your future efforts to reach Your Best Body more difficult! Today is the farthest you will ever be from Your Best Body. You will maintain Your Best Body for the long haul, as so many of my clients have, because you will have made realistic small changes, one day at a time, that add up to big results and simply become part of who you are.

Though you may begin the Countdown for one specific reason, you may discover it brings more benefits than you expected. Sonya is a wife, a mom of 3, and an elementary school principal in Augusta, Georgia. She completed the 52 day Countdown recently, losing 15 pounds of body fat while gaining strength and definition. After a couple weeks, she started the Countdown again and is down a total of about 30 pounds since she started the first round!

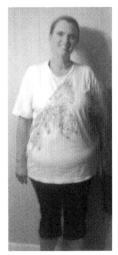 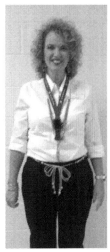 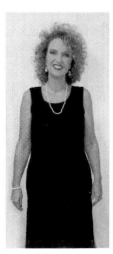

| Start of first 52-Day Countdown | End of first 52-Day Countdown | End of second 52-Day Countdown |

So, are you up for the challenge? I strongly suggest you use the Success Journal with a partner or a group for accountability and motivation. To get a jump start, you can read it straight through like a chapter book before you begin the 52 day Countdown. Or, simply read over tomorrow's challenge the day before, and set it out where you won't miss it at the start of your day! Fill in *all* the blanks and check off *every* box (meaning you completed that day's challenges). Plan to go through the 52 days again if needed, each time with more and more ease as you adapt to your healthy lifestyle — perhaps with a new partner that desires the results and freedom you will have achieved. I have found that progress is proportionate to the number of challenge boxes that are checked, and how many lines are filled.

The keys to my success with the 52 day countdown were filling half my plate at lunch and dinner with non-starchy veggies, tracking my food on an app, and exercising vigorously 5 days a week. I have never pushed my exercise to this level. I was motivated to exercise because I could eat more! I feel I can begin to see myself differently and I am proud of myself for meeting the fitness goals I set for myself. I want to model discipline and health for my kids and others I have influence over.

The keys to my success were...

Sonya, 47

Strength in numbers

Who do you know that wants to reach their Best Body too? You've heard there is strength in numbers, right? Accountability works! Don't go it alone. You need someone to encourage you when you want to give up, or even to compete with you. Who could go the 52-day distance with you?

- your spouse or close friend(s)
- your extended family
- your coworkers or worksite wellness group
- local gym members
- your singles group
- your local Mom's Club, preschool classroom moms or PTO
- your sports team or your kids' team parents
- your supper club
- your church during a church-wide health stewardship campaign
- your Sunday School class, Small Group, or Bible Study group

Please see Appendix A for a step-by-step guide for setting up a group to do the 52 Day Countdown with you!

Do you like to win?

Do you love a little competition or need some incentives to keep momentum strong? If so, talk with your partner, or your program coordinator/coach if you are doing the Countdown with a group, about what to do with the Best Body Ticket. There are 10 opportunities throughout the Countdown for you to earn a Best Body Ticket by simply showing your partner or coordinator/coach your progress on that day's challenges (see Appendix A). You may choose to drop a raffle ticket in a "hat" for each time a Best Body Ticket is earned and have a drawing at the end of the 52 days, or set up small rewards for each ticket earned for motivation along the way. Below are some prize ideas that promote wellness:

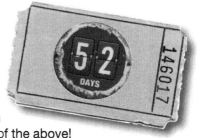

• gift card to a sports gear store
• gift card for a massage
• a new iPod
• iTunes gift card
• 3 or 6 month membership to a fitness facility
• a package with a personal trainer
• a consult with a registered dietitian
• a "Best Body Gift Basket" with all of the above!

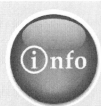

This 52 Day Countdown is not a substitute for a one-on-one consultation with a registered dietitian, as it is not customized to your individual needs. Registered dietitians (RDs or RDNs) are professionals who have earned a degree in nutrition and are required to stay abreast of ever-changing nutrition research in order to maintain RD or RDN status. If you have questions, a unique medical situation, or are in need of ongoing support, feel free to make an appointment with me for a personalized one-on-one nutrition consultation. I consult with clients for office appointments in the Augusta, Georgia area. For more information, check out bestbodyin52.com.

Or, visit eatright.org for a listing of registered dietitians near you. Best Bodies require diets that are based on the best available science and tailored to individual needs and circumstances by a professional who understands the biochemistry of the body. Use caution in taking recommendations from anyone who is not an RD/RDN or a licensed medical provider: much of my work is clean-up in the aftermath of poor advice.

Getting Started!

To get started on Your Best Body, you will need:

☑ an accountability/exercise partner
☑ comfortable athletic shoes
☑ an enticing water bottle/cup to use daily
☑ divided plates such as Chinet's disposable plates (check out preciseportions.com)
❑ optional: Gladware or Ziploc bowls in 1/2 cup and 1 cup servings (see Appendix J for food serving sizes)
☑ an exercise mat for outdoor exercise when and if applicable
☑ a pen and a highlighter for journaling your step-by-step success
❑ to complete the following "Kitchen Clean-up"
❑ to complete the Self-Assessment on page 30

13

"Kitchen Clean-Up"

If you can say YES to these, GREAT!

❏ Are most of your foods perishable?

❏ Do you have at least 3 rainbow colors of fresh fruit?

❏ Do you have veggies in at least 3 colors?

❏ Do you have any beans without sodium added?

❏ Do you have fish filets (frozen or fresh), or canned tuna or salmon?

❏ Are your meats lean cuts (skinless poultry, loin or round cuts for beef and pork, or >90% lean ground beef)?

❏ Are your dressings low or reduced fat?

❏ Are your cheeses low or reduced fat?

❏ Does your milk say Fat-Free (skim) or Reduced Fat (1%) on it (or your non-dairy alternative)?

❏ Are there any ready-to-serve healthy homemade leftovers in your freezer?

❏ Is there a tidy table where you can eat mindfully and without distraction?

❏ Do you have more whole grains than refined grains? Such as:

    ❏ Brown rice

    ❏ Oats

    ❏ Whole grain bread or pita

    ❏ Whole grain crackers/crispbreads

    ❏ Whole grain cereal

    ❏ Whole wheat pasta

❏ If I stopped by right now and looked in your pantry and fridge would I say "You are all set to reach Your Best Body!"?

If you answer YES to most of the following, it's time for a kitchen make-over!

❏ Are most of the items in your kitchen boxed or canned?

❏ Do the grains come with seasoning packets? (ex: Rice a Roni, Hamburger Helper)

❏ On the labels of your cereals and snacks, are added sugars listed as main ingredients (one of the first 3-5 listed)?

❏ Are many of your foods artificially flavored and colored?

❏ Are there foods that make your fingers feel greasy after eating?

❏ Do the ingredient lists include hydrogenated oils?

❏ Are there tempting snacks or sweets in plain view, or at your eye-level in the pantry or refrigerator?

❏ What about heavily processed or fatty meats like hot dogs, sausage, salami or bologna?

❏ Is salt the first ingredient of most of your spices/seasonings?

❏ Is your eating space one that directs your mind elsewhere while eating? (for example, cluttered with paperwork, or set up in front of the TV)

Don't miss this!

I will be using the following terms and phrases throughout your Success Journal. You may need to revisit this section if you find you have questions.

"REAL" water   8 | 8 oz glasses daily

Every day you will need to drink a minimum of 64 ounces of "REAL" water as part of the 52 day Countdown. It is unreasonable to think that your body can reach its best potential without meeting this most basic need. Water makes all the functions of your body work efficiently, promotes satiety, and prevents nagging headaches that slow you down. Think of it like the oil in your car...it doesn't make your car go, but even if you have a full tank of gas, without oil, you will not get anywhere.

By "REAL" water, I mean water without chemicals added. About half of your minimum of 64 ounces can be "sparkling" without additives (like La Croix), or you can add a couple of mini-ice cubes that you made from 100% juice. Water with fruit slices soaked in it overnight is perfect for those who dislike plain water. My favorite is water with sliced strawberries, cantaloupe, and oranges...it looks inviting, too! Try this: fill a pitcher with 64 ounces of water at night and add a few slices of various fresh fruits. By morning, your tinted "gourmet" water will be perfectly refreshing. Drink from that pitcher all day until it's empty and you have reached your daily goal of at least 64 ounces!

Does that seem like too much fluid for you? If taking in that much water is tough for you, then be sure to make the most of your thirst sensation! When exercising, or when you are hot or feeling thirsty, don't just take a few sips, but finish off at least a large glass or bottle of water.

I always make sure I finish at least one water bottle during exercise, and then another on the ride home from the gym.

Tea you make with hot water and a tea bag (without sugar added) can also count towards your "REAL" water goal. My favorite is herbal peppermint tea. Chilled or hot, it's very refreshing, even with no sweetener. You can also fill a water pitcher with fresh mint leaves and ice for a similar taste. If you are used to drinking caloric beverages, many of which are loaded with additives and sweeteners, it won't hurt you one bit if you find you just don't have room to fit them in on top of your 64 ounces of "REAL" water!

"Move"

Of the National Weight Control Registry members who have lost an average of 66 pounds and kept it off for 5.5 years (impressive!), 90% report doing about an hour of exercise daily. Ninety-eight percent of Registry participants report that they modified their food intake as well. Your health goals, and weight loss or maintenance aspirations will not likely be met without a combination of both exercise and changes to improve your diet.

When you see "move" in this Success Journal, I mean a total of about an hour of movement that increases your heart rate and respiration, and typically causes light to heavy perspiration, depending on the intensity level. That said, we are going to categorize half of the time (about half an hour) as casual to moderate intensity (think "Don't just stand there, move!"), and the other half as moderately intense to intense activity (think "Move it! Move it!"). Our Best Body goal: MOVE for 52 minutes (about an hour) 5 days per week. Don't worry. You'll see that it's more feasible than you think.

Doing both kinds of movement over the course of your day will promote an active, flexible lifestyle that can be maintained rather than just adhered to for a few weeks. I ask you do both because I want you not only to burn a bunch of calories to create that calorie deficit needed for weight control, but also to mobilize those free fatty acids that are more likely to be burned up at a lower intensity. In short, just put on comfortable shoes for movement until you are in bed for the night, and make sure about half an hour sets you up for a shower. If casual movement is intense for you, then just try your best to accumulate 52 minutes of movement before the day ends. Everyone has to start somewhere! The less time you spend on your couch, the better!

"Move it! Move it!"

In order to put a check in the "move for 52 minutes" box you'll see throughout the Countdown, at least half of the 52 minutes must be intense (think "Move it! Move it!" for about a half hour). If you rate your perceived exertion on a scale of 1-10, you should be working at a 6.5 to 9 intensity during that "Move it! Move it" portion of your daily exercise. Though you should be able to speak (not sing), having a conversation while exercising should be challenging for those minutes. Examples of this type of exercise include the "Take Tens" you'll find in the Success Journal, aerobics classes where you leave fully spent, interval style workouts such as high intensity interval training (HIIT), lap swimming, jogging/running, playing basketball, cycling, and heavy weight lifting with very short rest-breaks. If you're just beginning, you may be at that intensity level with much less rigorous exercise and that's okay.

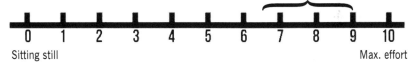

"Don't just stand there, move!"

For the less intense half-hour (think, "Don't just stand there, move!"), you should feel your heart rate elevated, and have at least light perspiration by the time 10 minutes accumulate. On a scale of 1-10, your intensity level should be about 4 - 6.5. This is casual to moderately intense movement like brisk walking, yard-work, recreational swimming, quick-paced vacuuming/mopping, golfing without a cart, light/moderate weight lifting, yoga, a leisurely bike ride, or walking up stairs.

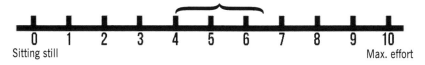

You can check off your "Move for 52 minutes" box if you:
"Move it! Move it!" for about a half hour
AND
"Don't just stand there, Move!" for about a half hour.

According to the American
College of Sports Medicine, research shows that 10-minute
bouts of exercise are effective when they accumulate daily,
so keep in mind that your exercise does not have to be for 52
consecutive minutes. What great news for those who don't feel
they have an hour to spare! However, if you know that doing
these short bouts will prevent you from pushing yourself to
do higher intensity exercises, especially as your fitness level
increases, please save these 10-minute bouts for your lower
intensity segments of exercise.

Make it work for you! Below are some examples that you can do to
check off your exercise for the day:

○ an hour-long interval aerobics class

○ a half hour cardio DVD workout in the morning before showering,
and a family bike-ride in the evening

○ golfing without a cart for 18 holes and moving as briskly as
possible...adding up to about 25-30 minutes of intense movement
(pulling cart uphill) and 30+ of moderately intense movement

○ "Mommy and me" or "Daddy and me" hour at the park: active play
with your toddler at the park for 25 minutes, and then getting out the
stroller for a very brisk walk/jog for the other half

○ a high intensity interval training workout for 30 minutes with your
partner and gardening later in the day

○ briskly walking the halls at work for 10-minute bouts twice during
the workday, and later stopping by the gym for heavy weight lifting (with
short rest breaks so your heart rate stays up)

I'm a stay-at-home mom with three boys
ages 5 and under. Instead of
showering first thing and getting
dressed for the day, while doing
the 52 day Countdown, I learned
to just start the morning in
exercise clothes and tennis shoes
and make the most of every 10-
minute opportunity to be active
with the children until I had
reached 52 minutes.

**Make the most of every
10-minute opportunity.**

Bianca, 39

○ walking "hills" very briskly on your treadmill during the evening news (30 minutes) and doing a yoga video before bed to finish out the 52 minutes

○ two "Take Tens" (see Appendix I) before showering in the morning, and shoot hoops with your children after work for about half an hour

○ taking a walk with a friend on your lunch-break, and attending a 30 minute Boot Camp class later that evening

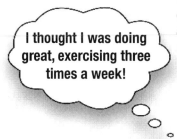

I thought I was doing great, exercising three times a week!

You most certainly are! However, our bodies were intended to move a lot more than they do in a typical, often sedentary twenty-first century day. The American College of Sports Medicine (the gold standard for exercise guidelines) makes the following recommendation for maintaining *general* good health. (In other words, this is not the recommendation for those with high cholesterol, high blood pressure, or those who are overweight or obese. Those conditions may require more time, and require consultation with a physician.)

Exercise guidelines from the American College of Sports Medicine and the American Heart Association

Do moderately intense cardio 30 minutes a day, 5 days/wk
Or
Do vigorously intense cardio 20 minutes a day, 3 days/wk
And
Do 8 to 10 strength-training exercises, 8 to 12 repetitions of each exercise twice a week.

·Moderate-intensity physical activity means working hard enough to raise your heart rate and break a sweat, yet still being able to carry on a conversation.

·To lose weight or maintain weight loss, 60 to 90 minutes of physical activity may be necessary.

·The 30-minute recommendation is for the average healthy adult to maintain health and reduce the risk for chronic disease.

My recommendation of about an hour of exercise 5 days a week is to help you reach Your Best Body. If you are already healthy and lean, your calories are under control daily, and you are not needing to lose weight or combat any chronic conditions, you can follow the 3-5 day guidelines just noted, adding the strength training if you have not yet done so. However, be sure to prioritize casual to moderate movement whenever you can outside of those 3-5 planned workouts!

Once you have achieved your healthy weight goal and your fitness level, general activity level, and overall diet have improved, you can go from the hour to about half of that, as noted in the American College of Sports Medicine (ACSM) guidelines (p. 19). This decrease in time works assuming you will be more fit and can push yourself harder in a shorter amount of time. And you will be more likely to burn calories throughout the day due to greater ease in movement and increases in lean body mass. Keep in mind, however, ACSM does state that to lose or maintain weight loss, 60 to 90 minutes of physical activity may be necessary. The amount of time you need to spend burning calories largely depends on your calorie intake as well.

Myth:

Exercise causes weight loss.

Fact:

A calorie deficit is needed for weight loss. (You will learn more about this throughout the Countdown.)

To protect yourself from injury, you need to be mindful of any limitations you have when beginning an exercise program or taking your current activity to the next level. Talk to your healthcare provider about any precautions you should take and get clearance to begin regular exercise. (If weight loss is your goal, as you lose weight, you will likely need to reduce some medications, particularly those for blood pressure and blood sugar management, so stay in touch with your medical care provider.) Though you may be eager to get started, overdoing exercise at the start of a new program may not only cause injury, but delay your progress due to immobility from soreness and tight muscles.

Flexibly also is key to injury prevention. Take time to warm up and cool down for 5-10 minutes at the start and finish of activity. Hold stretches for major muscle groups for 30 seconds at the end of your exercise time when your muscles are nice and warm. Be careful not to overtrain, keeping in mind that a major injury may set you back farther than your initial Countdown starting point.

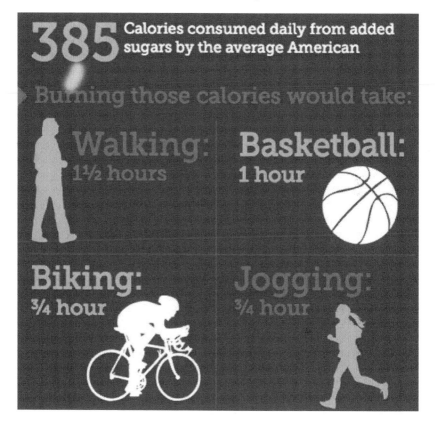

385 Calories consumed daily from added sugars by the average American

Burning those calories would take:

Walking: 1½ hours

Basketball: 1 hour

Biking: ¾ hour

Jogging: ¾ hour

"Added Sugar"

When the challenges mention avoiding added sugar, I mean any sugars other than those that occur naturally in whole foods. These sugars are added during processing or preparation. Naturally occurring sugars such as those coming from plain milk and fruit do not count toward your added sugar total. If there is a gram of sugar in your plain old-fashioned oats, for example, that is not because it's been added (so that is okay). But, if your cereal has honey or evaporated cane juice, or if your snacks have dextrose, high fructose corn syrup, or brown sugar, those grams will count as added sugar.

Your food label will list the "sugars" in grams, but be aware that the number of grams listed is the sum of both naturally occurring sugars and added sugar, which can make mixed foods difficult to figure out without reading the ingredient list. The following graphic from the Center for Science in the Public Interest shows the foods and beverages to watch out for. Notice that the main culprit is not the teaspoon of sugar you add to your coffee, but rather the beverages, snacks, and desserts that are sweetened before you even purchase them.

Why limit added sugars? Not only are the estimated 385 calories from added sugars that Americans average daily amounting to extra weight, they are leading to illnesses that take us far from our Best

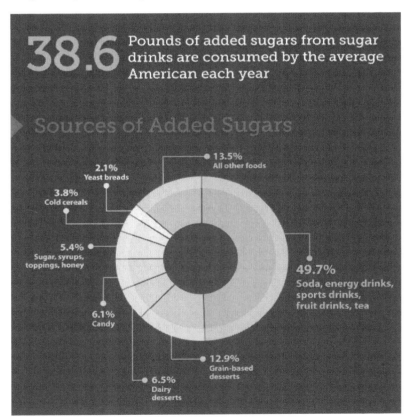

Body aspirations! And, if consumed, those daily sugar calories are just barely burned off during your daily exercise goal of 52 minutes. The challenges regarding added sugar throughout this Success Journal will help you stay within the recommendations set by the American Heart Association.

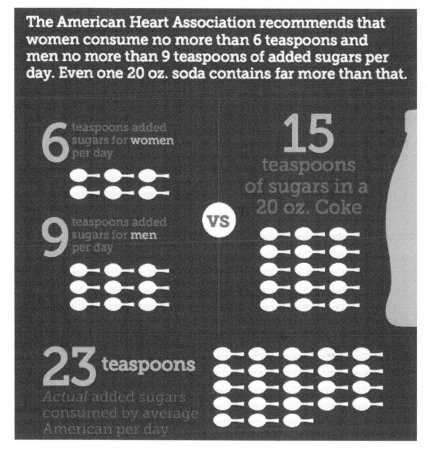

The American Heart Association recommends that women consume no more than 6 teaspoons and men no more than 9 teaspoons of added sugars per day. Even one 20 oz. soda contains far more than that.

6 teaspoons added sugars for **women** per day

9 teaspoons added sugars for **men** per day

VS

15 teaspoons of sugars in a 20 oz. Coke

23 teaspoons
Actual added sugars consumed by average American per day

You will achieve Your Best Body more quickly if you avoid added sugars as much as possible.

Pounds and Calories

Questions about pounds and calories always arise, whether doing the Countdown to Your Best Body for weight loss, to make an impact on a specific health concern, or to find out what life is like when your body is at its best.

How often should I weigh?

I suggest weighing only once a week from here on out. Weigh at the same time of day after using the restroom, at the same level of hydration, and in the same type of clothing. Please see the Appendix B and C for a graph on which to record your weekly weight.

What should I weigh?

If you have read this far, then you know you need to make some changes to reach Your Best Body. Whether a chart suggests that you are "overweight" or "obese" will not affect your progress in the Countdown. To determine what you should weigh, consider your health indicators (labs, etc.) and your weight over the past 5 years. Aim for the weight you were when you were most healthy according to your medical chart and when you felt your best. When you reach it, reassess considering your health and risk factors, and how you feel about yourself. I am not putting a Body Mass Index (BMI) or weight chart in this Success Journal - telling you the exact number of pounds you should weigh. Though they are helpful for assessing general populations, for most people, they stir up more frustration than motivation.

However, understanding the risks related to the composition of your weight may motivate you to do your very best over the next 52 days, and those following. If your waist circumference is greater than 35 inches for women, and 40 inches for men, you are at greater risk for several serious conditions responsible for premature death and diminishing quality of life: high blood pressure, type 2 diabetes, coronary artery disease, high cholesterol, and metabolic syndrome. Your waist circumference will improve with the exercise regimen and diet changes suggested in this Countdown, provided you are not taking in more calories than you are burning.

What about calorie counting?

Calories certainly do count, so in order to reach Your Best Body, you must consider their coming and going: your calorie balance equation. If you have dieted or committed to exercise before, you may have found that calorie-management can be frustrating, to say the least. Add to that the mixed messages you get from different websites' calorie goals for you, and you'll just end up wasting your 52 minutes of "move" time surfing the internet and not getting concrete answers.

For years I have heard people say, "Just tell me exactly what to do and I will just do it. Tell me what to eat exactly, and I will just eat that." As much as I would like to make it that simple, you know if you have ever tried a diet that tells you exactly what to eat each day, that you won't stick with it for long. Every "Best Body in-the-making" is unique. The math of calories taken in (food and drink) and burned off (exercise and daily body functions) matters, but it is not to be your focus as you work towards Your Best Body. I have done the "accounting" work for you behind the scenes to save you from obsessing over the numbers. I am not going to go into all the details of how your metabolism works, though fascinating; I am just going to tell you what you need to know to get started, and give you more details and reminders throughout the 52 days of the Countdown.

To explain your caloric needs, I will present my "Smart Car vs. Expedition" analogy. When I was a college student at the University of Georgia, I drove a small car. Not only did it have a small engine thus requiring very little gas, but I didn't have to do a lot of driving around Athens as a student. Fast forward 15 years to me as a soccer Mom with a loaded down Ford Expedition. Not only is it a bigger engine, but there is a lot more coming and going. Your "fuel" needs (that is, your caloric needs) will depend on the size of your "engine" (your lean body mass), and how much time you spend "on the road" (moving and exercising). The amount of "fuel" you need is different than that of your spouse or roommate, and may even be different than it was last year.

> Your "fuel" needs (that is, your caloric needs), will depend on the size of your "engine" (your lean body mass), and how much time you spend "on the road" (moving and exercising).

To consider how much fuel you need to "put in your tank," let's go through some of the questions I ask in consultations to assess my client's caloric needs.

Circle the kind of "car" you drive.

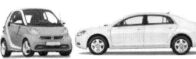

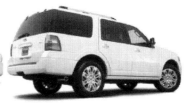

Petite frame,
non-muscular
build

Average build,
average muscle
mass

Large frame,
muscular build

Now let's talk about what kind of "driver" you are.
Circle the kind of driver you are:

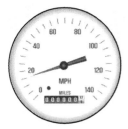

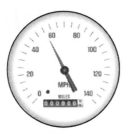

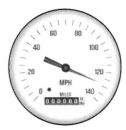

When I move,
I move slowly.

Average. I move,
but I don't set any
speed records.

I move with the
pedal to the
metal.

Carrying on with the analogy, you also must consider how often and how far you drive, so to speak, when you do get on the road. Check which one of these best describes you. (This is not taking into account intentional exercise).

❑ "People are always trying to keep up with me when I am walking throughout my day, often telling me to slow down."

❑ "I am constantly moving, bending, and lifting at work or at home."

❑ "I am on my feet most of the day, but am mostly standing still when I am up."

❑ "I am in a desk or chair most of the day."

Imagine automatically putting ten gallons of gas in your actual car every day, even if you don't do much driving. Consider how that analogy applies to you. If you fill your body's tank but don't do a lot of driving, when you refuel again the fuel will "spill out" (that is, overflow into fat storage). Try to spend more time "on the road" than you do "at the station." Also when fueling, keep in mind what kind of car you drive and how far you will be driving that day.

The bottom line: most people should move a lot more and eat a little less! For the majority of adults, the calories needed to maintain weight are typically anywhere from 1200 to 2500 per day, depending on the factors previously mentioned. To lose 1-2 pounds per week, reduce your caloric intake by 250-500 per day, and exercise to burn an extra 250-500 calories. The total weekly deficit of 3500-7000 calories leads to 1-2 pounds of fat loss, respectively. Men and

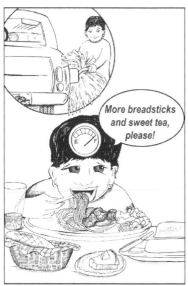

Graphic from Edna Harris-Davis.
Used with permission.

women needing to lose weight typically need to eat between 1200-1800 calories daily. Again, whether you need 1200 or 1800, or somewhere in between depends on how much lean tissue you have, and your activity level.

The final consideration in this analogy is the type or grade of fuel. Many of my clients think that since they use "premium fuel" (healthy food), they can fuel up as often as they like. However, even healthy food can cause an overflow of "fuel" into your fat cells to be stored as fat tissue. It's all about the balance. You will learn more about each of these factors over the next 52 days. Review the serving sizes and a sample day's menu on the next two pages to get an idea of where to start.

excess fuel = fat tissue
(even if it's premium grade fuel)

inadequate fuel =
compromised metabolism

Serving Sizes

Hint: 1 grain or starch = 15 g carb; limit or avoid those along the bottom

Meats	Vegetables	Grain/Starch	Fruit	Dairy	Fat
Fish (not fried) Salmon, trout, herring, flounder, mackerel, tuna, and others	1 cup raw vegetables ½ cup cooked or finely chopped vegetables	1/3 cup cooked rice	1 tennis ball-sized fruit such as an apple, peach, etc.	1 cup skim or 1% milk	2 tbsp. avocado (1/5) 8 olives
Poultry: White meat, no skin	starchy vegetables and beans are counted with grains because of their starchy quality	1/2 cup cooked pasta, oats, quinoa, bulgur, or barley	½ banana	1 cup yogurt, regular or Greek yogurt	4–10 nuts 1 ½ tsp nut butter 1 tbsp. sunflower, pumpkin, or flax seeds
Beef and Pork: Loin and round cuts are typically lean		½ cup grits	¾ cup any berries	1.5 oz fat-free or reduced-fat cheese Mozzarella, ricotta, and feta are naturally lower in fat	1 tsp. oil 1 tbsp. Promise or Smart Balance spread
lean lunch meat (limit nitrates) 1 egg = 1 oz. meat		6 saltine-size crackers or 2 crisp-breads	1 cup any melon cubes		1 tbsp. salad dressing (2 if tbsp. light)
		1 slice whole-grain bread (1 ounce)	½ cup applesauce, unsweetened	¼ cup low-fat cottage cheese	2 tsp. mayo 1 tsp. coconut oil 1 tsp. butter 1 tbsp. cream cheese
		½ whole wheat pita or English muffin	2 tbsp. dried fruits		
		¾ cup whole-grain cereal	4 ounces 100% juice		
		1/2 cup of corn, peas, potatoes, sweet potatoes, or beans			
Avoid: Bologna, bacon, sausage, salami, hot dogs, and limit highly processed deli meats		Limit: White or refined grain products, biscuits, cornbread, granola, fried potatoes, waffles, cookies, and cakes	Limit: Juice, fruit drinks	Limit: Whole milk, full-fat cheeses and yogurts, ice cream, cream soups	Limit or Avoid: Butter, cream soups, stick margarine, bacon, fatback, gravy, cream, shortening, full-fat dressings, and hydrogenated oils (trans fat) in packaged products

"Fueling" for Your Best Body

Sample Day

This sample day is about 1600 calories. See a registered dietitian to customize your calorie level, as 1600 calories is not appropriate for all.

Breakfast: 7 AM
black coffee (sweeten with Stevia or Splenda if needed)
1 cup of fat free or 1% milk (to drink, or mix in oatmeal or coffee)
1/2 cup cooked old fashioned oatmeal with 1/2 teaspoon brown sugar added
1 slice of whole wheat toast with 1 1/2 teaspoons peanut butter
1 orange, whole (or choose another fruit to mix into oatmeal)
water

10:30 AM: 1 apple and sparkling water with no additives

Lunch: 12:00 PM
3 ounces of tuna with 1 1/2 teaspoons light mayo, add 1/2 cup of finely chopped raw spinach and stir it in (try the food processor to chop)
4 Ryvita Sesame Rye crisp-bread crackers
1 cup Refreshing Rainbow Salad (see Day 51 for recipe)
water

"Strong Snack:" 3:30 PM
8 ounces (1 cup) unsweetened Greek yogurt with 3/4 cup mixed blueberries and strawberries and 1/2 teaspoon honey if needed
6 almonds
hot or chilled peppermint tea, unsweetened

Dinner: 6:30 PM
Perfectly Filling Lettuce Wraps (see Day 40 for recipe)
3 1/2 ounce chicken breast, marinated in The Perfect Dressing (see Day 47 for recipe)
unsweetened tea with lemon

Self Assessment

Date: ....

On a scale of 1-5 (1 being "not at all likely," and 5 being "definitely"), what is the likelihood that you will make the following commitments daily for the next 52 days:

Complete each day's challenges and fill in answers to the questions:	Stay committed to my partner/this program for 52 days.	Exercise for 52 minutes, 5 days a week (about half of which is intense):
1 2 3 4 5	1 2 3 4 5	1 2 3 4 5

I am not beautiful like you,
I'm beautiful like me.
Anonymous

Before Reaching Your Best Body

Name:	Date:
Accountability Partner:	
Weight:	Height:
Waist circumference measurement: ....inches *Measure around the smallest part of the waist while standing relaxed.*	
Measurement in one other location where you tend to put on weight/fat (where exactly: ....and inches:...........)	
Maximum number of seconds you can hold a plank with good form (assessed by someone else):	

The Front Plank

Step 1
Starting Position:
Lie flat on your stomach with your elbows tucked in at your sides, palms down. Engage your core muscles as if you are pressing your naval to your spine. It should feel as if someone is tightening a corset around your core from your ribs to your hips. Contract your thigh muscles to make your legs straight and strong. Flex your ankles, tucking your toes toward your shins.

Step 2
Upward Phase:
Slowly lift your upper body and thighs off the floor. Keep your legs and torso rigid. Do not let your ribcage or hips drop or sag. Conversely, do not hike your hips into the air or bend your knees. Make sure your shoulders do not shrug toward your ears. The shoulders need to be directly over your elbows with your palms facing down. Hold the positing while breathing normally and keeping the abdominals engaged. Try to hold this plank position as long as possible with good form.

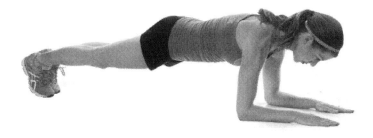

Step 3
Downward Phase:
Lower gently back to the floor while keeping your torso and legs stiff. If you have acute lower back pain, do not continue with this exercise until you have consulted with your doctor.

Day 52

Just me! Date: _____

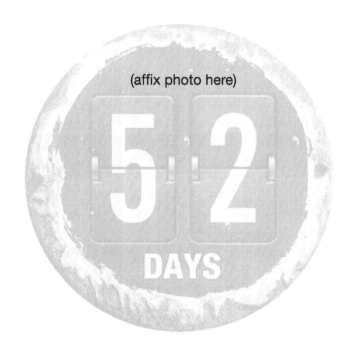

(affix photo here)

My partner and me! Date: _____

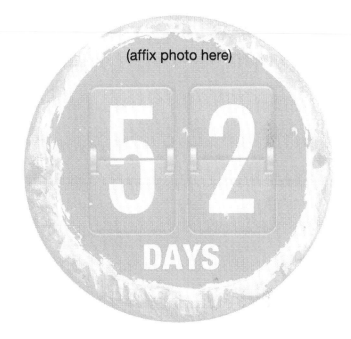

(affix photo here)

Day 24

I'm halfway there!
Just me! Date: _____

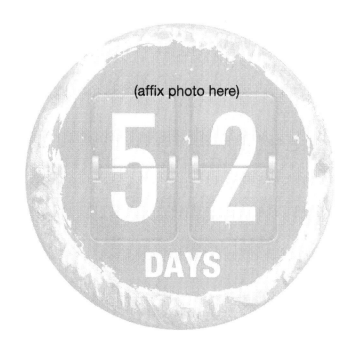

(affix photo here)

52 DAYS

My partner and me! Date: _____

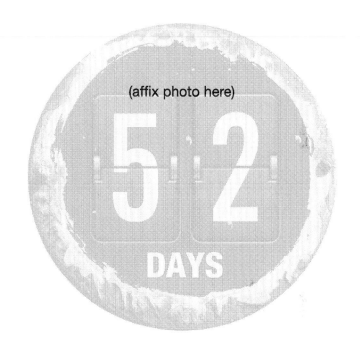

(affix photo here)

Day 1

I made it 52 days!
Just me! Date: _____

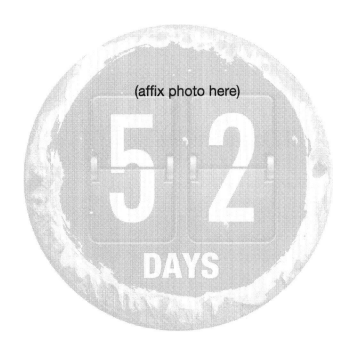

(affix photo here)

My partner and me! Date: _____

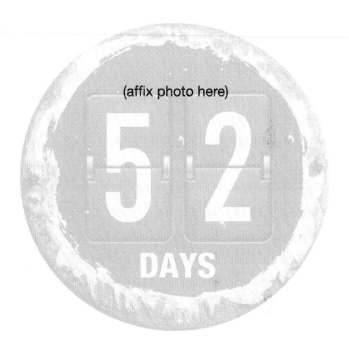

(affix photo here)

Are you Ready?

You know you really can -
You can stay focused for 52 days!
You CAN reach Your Best Body!
You will truly be amazed!

Astounded by your own progress,
Your leanness and self-control
(No need to suck in, and goodbye Spanx),
Energized as you meet your goals!

But, that means no excuses...
That's right, even if they are reasonable.
With 1248 hours to do it,
What the Countdown requires IS feasible.

I'm asking you to think before you act,
To plan a little and prioritize;
To put your health before your urges-
Knowing the price is worth the prize!

Ignore the contradicting messages.
Avoid comparison and magazines,
Instead zone in on each challenge
To ensure your success is felt and seen.

I know what it takes to reach your Best Body:
The attitude: "for 52 days - I must!"
Plus accountability and this Journal
(well sure, new kicks are a plus).

Driven by despised humps and bumps?
I get it - you want those gone.
But I've got your lean lifetime in mind:
Inside and out - lifelong strong!

So look your partner in the eyes
And say, "we CAN do this, you and me!
Let's move a lot more and eat a little less.
Let the Countdown begin...WE ARE READY!"

"Don't be afraid your life will end;
be afraid that it will never begin."

-Grace Hansen

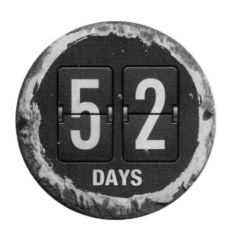

The 52 Day Countdown

For 52 days, mark off as many of the check-boxes as you can, indicating that you have completed the daily steps to reaching Your Best Body. Make it a priority to fill in every line and check every box.

The quotes and frequently asked questions (FAQs) throughout this Success Journal are from my clients and others who have worked through the daily Best Body challenges you are about to begin. They have given me permission to share a part of their journey with you. They would agree with me that if you start strong, and stay committed, you will finish at your BEST.

Day 52

❑ Drink 64+ ounces of "REAL" water (no chemicals added).
❑ Move for 52 minutes (at least half must be intense - meaning you are working at a 6.5 to 9 on scale of 1-10 for about half an hour). Mark your exercise daily in the "Move for 52 Minutes Log" in Appendix D to keep track of your exercise progress in one place.
❑ Consume no more than 5 grams of added sugar daily (see label for "sugars") from food or beverages - just for 7 days! That is just about 1 teaspoon, so spend it wisely! Sugars naturally occurring in fruit and plain milk are not added sugars, so they are okay, in moderation, of course. Refer back to pages 21 through 23 for information regarding added sugar versus sugar naturally occurring in foods.

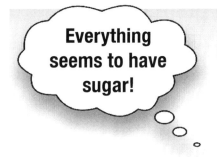

Everything seems to have sugar!

"I've been checking labels to get ready for the Countdown, and everything seems to have sugar! The only way I know to go without added sugar this week is just to eat basics like veggies, meat, and potatoes."

Regan, 34

❏ Take a picture in fitted workout clothes, standing with your accountability partner (game-faces of course!).

❏ Also, take a photo of each other. You might dread doing this, but you will be glad you did at the half-way point, and as you are counting down from Day 52 to Day 1. Seeing your progress is motivating!

❏ Print and affix your photos in the designated place in the previous section of this journal.

Write 52 things you'll be thrilled about when you reach Your Best Body! Think not only about your looks, your self-confidence, and how you'll feel in your clothes, but how it will impact your long term health, your future finances, your family, your work, and your social life.

Ideas:
• It will feel good to be me.
• I will be off cholesterol meds!
• I will be a good example to my children.
• I will be spending my money on active fun rather than on clothes that are the next size up.
• My significant other will be amazed!

1-...
2-...
3-...
4-...
5-...
6-...
7-...
8-...
9-...
10-...
11-...
12-...
13-...
14-...
15-...
16-...
17-...

18-..
19-..
20-..
21-..
22-..
23-..
24-..
25-..
26-..
27-..
28-..
29-..
30-..
31-..
32-..
33-..
34-..
35-..
36-..
37-..
38-..
39-..
40-..
41-..
42-..
43-..
44-..
45-..
46-..
47-..
48-..
49-..
50-..
51-..
52-..

"It was really tough to think of 52. I filled out about half of it, and then came back to it at the end of the day, but I did fill in all 52 lines!"

Maria, 29

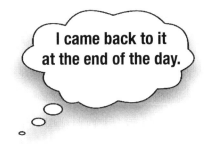

I came back to it at the end of the day.

Day 51

❑ Drink 64+ ounces of "REAL" water (no chemicals added).

❑ Move for 52 minutes (at least half must be intense - meaning you are working at a 6.5 to 9 on scale of 1-10 for about half an hour). Mark your exercise daily in the "Move for 52 Minutes Log" in Appendix D to keep track of your exercise progress all in one place.

❑ Consume no more than 5 grams of added sugar daily (see label for "sugars") from food or beverages - just for 6 more days! Remember, that is just about 1 teaspoon. Sugars naturally occurring in fruit and plain milk are okay in moderation.

FAQ

Q: "What about yogurt?" It seems to have a lot of sugar. I was disappointed to find out that my normal breakfast of Greek yogurt and granola would put me over the daily maximum for sugar.

Ashley, 28

A: Sugar that naturally occurs in milk and fruit is not considered "added" sugar. Yogurt is tricky because the "sugars" on the label can be from both naturally occurring sugars (the milk sugar, lactose, and the fruit sugar, fructose) as well as added sugars. In 6 ounces of plain yogurt, there are about 12 grams of naturally occurring lactose sugar, and no added sugar. Ideally eat the plain kind and add fruit to sweeten it healthfully. On average, fruit-flavored yogurt has an additional 10-14 grams of sugar from added fruit and sweeteners combined. Light yogurts typically use sugar-substitutes to cut back on sugar and calories. I am conservative in my use of artificial sweeteners, encouraging clients to max out at about one to two servings of artificially sweetened food and beverages daily. Yogurt has many benefits that make it a worthwhile daily choice, even if means you avoid a diet drink later in the day in order to limit artificial sweetener intake. Greek yogurt has even more protein to hold you over to your next meal, and naturally less sugar (from lactose, which means those who are lactose intolerant can tolerate small amounts of Greek yogurt better). But, it also has a little less calcium than regular yogurt. My recommendation: add fruit and nuts to Fat Free Plain Greek yogurt. The following give you the most calcium and protein for 100 calories: Dannon Oikos, Chobani, Brown Cow, Fage, Skyr, Smári, and Wallaby Organic.

Time for a "detox!" It's probably not what you are thinking. I would not suggest anyone exercise intensely while going through the lethargy and abdominal distress that accompany a typical detox. If you eat according to the guidelines in this book, you will see that you do not have the need for that type of detox.

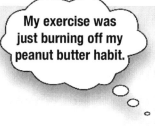

My exercise was just burning off my peanut butter habit.

I was in the habit of walking into my apartment after work, getting a big spoon and going straight for the peanut butter. Then I'd go for a run. Eventually I realized my exercise was pretty much just burning off my peanut butter habit. So, I switched to natural peanut butter which was just as good on a sandwich, but didn't tempt me to get a heaping spoonful.

Me, at 22

☐ This "detox" will help you to eliminate a total of at least 10 things from your life that you suspect are not promoting your success! Think about what or who makes you feel unsuccessful or out of control, or drains your confidence. Thinking through this might prompt you to sit down and share your health goals and your new boundaries with anyone on the "discouragers" list. Or, perhaps you can identify "trigger" foods to which you can't seem to say no. Determine that these are not welcome in your eyeshot for at least 51 days. Feel free at that point to reassess, but you may find it is just not wise to reintroduce known hinderances of your success.

FOODS AND BEVERAGES	SHOWS, MAGAZINES OR WEBSITES	HABITS	DISCOURAGERS
Examples: wine/beer, chocolate, cheese, chips, peanut butter.	Magazines that make me focus too much on my flaws.	Eating while watching TV. Always holding a drink.	My co-worker who always brings cookies.

Refreshing Rainbow Salad

Serves 6

1/2 bag (about 6 ounces) rainbow slaw
(also called California slaw or broccoli slaw)
1 Granny Smith apple, washed and cored, with peel
1/2 cup golden raisins
1/2 cup slivered almonds
2 teaspoons lemon juice

1. Briefly pulse rainbow slaw and apple together in a food processor or blender until coarsely chopped. Place in a large bowl.
2. Add the lemon juice, almonds, and raisins. Toss and serve promptly.

Nutrient Breakdown: Calories 127, Fat 5g, Carb 19 g, Fiber 7 g, Sodium 12 mg, Sugar 4 g (all from fruit, so none is considered added sugar)

Day 50

❏ Drink 64+ ounces of "REAL" water (no chemicals added).

❏ Move for 52 minutes (at least half must be intense - meaning you are working at a 6.5 to 9 on scale of 1-10 for about half an hour).

❏ Consume no more than 5 grams of added sugar daily (see label for "sugars") from food or beverages - just for 5 more days!

Now that you have noted some things you should avoid, what should you put on your plate?

❏ Fill half of your plate with non-starchy veggies at lunch and dinner (2-3 servings). That leaves about a quarter of your plate for lean protein, and the other quarter for starches, whole grains and starchy vegetables. Add a thumb tip serving of fat and your plate is set up for success. Visualize your foods fitting into this compartmentalized plate, keeping in mind that how much you should put in each section is based on the car analogy I shared with you previously. Consider eating from a plate divided like the one pictured below. (Visit preciseportions.com for options. They also carry compostable divided plates, or you can get some Chinet plates at your grocery store to get started.)

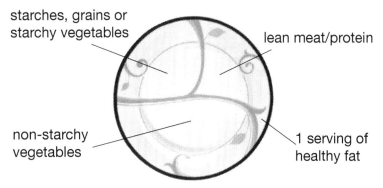

starches, grains or starchy vegetables

lean meat/protein

non-starchy vegetables

1 serving of healthy fat

Prioritizing your vegetables is one of the best things you can commit to doing from now on, and even beyond this Countdown. These tasty "go-withs" help to fill you up for very few calories, not to mention their powerful antioxidants and chronic disease-fighting potential. Not only are they good for you, but they protect you from the alternative: what would you be putting on half of your plate if not non-starchy vegetables?

In the South, we have two main vegetables: green beans (often cooked in grease) and iceberg lettuce drenched in ranch dressing. Perhaps it's time to branch out and view vegetables from a new perspective. They will be deserving of much of the credit for your Best Body if you give them the chance. They don't have to be a pile of mush on your plate that you dread having to choke down. For recipes and meal plans that set your plate up for success, check out my website (bestbodyin52.com).

Try not just to recall what you don't like about certain veggies. I've learned it's all about how they are prepared, and often when mixed into something delicious, or in a new recipe, you won't mind them one bit. Simply stand in the produce section and look around at your options: perhaps there are some vegetables you have dismissed which deserve another chance...maybe this time prepared an entirely different way, and consumed with a smile. Like I tell my kids, "Of course food tastes bad if you frown while you are eating it." Take this seriously - your success at becoming more lean and healthy largely depends on the make-up of half your plate!

Consider the vegetables listed below in a new light. Some preparation suggestions for non-starchy veggies include steaming, roasting, grilling, and stir-frying; or add to soups, salads, sandwiches and casseroles.

Artichokes	Celery	Onions
Asparagus	Cucumber	Peppers
Green Beans	Eggplant	Snow Peas
Beets	Garlic	Spinach
Broccoli	Greens, various	Squash, various
Brussels sprouts	Leeks	Tomatoes
Cabbage	Lettuce	Zucchini
Carrots	Mushrooms	
Cauliflower	Okra	

Until I grew eggplant in my backyard, I was convinced I didn't like it. I figured if I grew it, perhaps I would experiment enough to learn how I liked it. It worked! Try the following sandwich, even if you dislike eggplant. It's the perfect combination of flavors and is a favorite to even the most devout meat-lovers in my family.

Toasted Eggplant Sandwiches

Serves 4

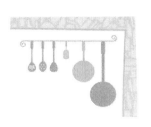

1 small eggplant, peeled and thinly sliced
2 tsp olive oil, or use cooking spray/oil
1/2 cup light mayonnaise
3 cloves of garlic, minced
8 whole wheat pita halves, unopened, or 4
sandwich "thins" (whole wheat)
2 tomatoes, sliced
1/2 cup crumbled feta cheese
1/4 cup fresh basil leaves, chopped

1. Preheat oven to 400 degrees. Lightly spray eggplant slices with olive oil (from a spray bottle or cooking spray) and place them on a baking sheet. Place pan about 6" from the heat source. Cook for 10 minutes or until tender and toasted.
2. Lightly toast the pita in the oven (about 2 minutes). In a small bowl, stir together the mayo, garlic and basil. Spread mixture on the toasted pita/bread. Layer with eggplant, tomato, and feta cheese.

Nutrient Breakdown: Calories 342, Fat 18 g,
Carb 39 g, Fiber 7 g, Protein 9 g

Pair this with cup of Greek yogurt for dessert to bump up the total protein since it's a meatless meal.

Day 49

❏ Drink 64+ ounces of "REAL" water (no chemicals added).
❏ Consume no more than 5 grams of added sugar daily (see label for "sugars") from food or beverages - just for 4 more days!
❏ Fill half of your plate with non-starchy veggies at lunch and dinner (2-3 servings).
❏ Move for 52 minutes, but here are the rules of play:
❏ Three times today, do the following "Take Ten" exercise. This ten-minute full body workout is meant to be challenging for every fitness level. You wouldn't expect to reach Your Best Body with anything less, would you? Just do your best and take short breaks if needed. If you are already conditioned to intense exercise, then add weight to the exercises that apply to make them more challenging.

If you plan to do this "Take Ten" three times back to back, get together with your partner for motivation and encouragement! This will be your intense exercise segment for today, working at an intensity level of 6.5 - 9 on a scale of 1 - 10. Keep in mind this looks different for everyone. There will be a few more "Take Tens" throughout the Countdown.

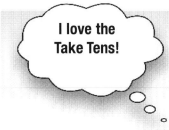

I love the Take Tens!

I love the "Take Tens." You can easily do them at home or out of town to get a quick workout in. They are challenging and fun to do with a friend.

Dena, 42

If needed, see http://www.acefitness. org/acefit/exercise-library-main/ for proper form of any of the following Take Ten exercises, typing the name of the exercise with the asterisk in the search bar.

Take Ten

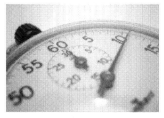

Minute 1: hold a plank (this will warm you up; see page 31 for instructions)
Minute 2: bodyweight squats* - hips level with knees before rising back up
Minute 3: 30 seconds of push-ups, 30 seconds of triceps dips
Minute 4: dance like you know you are a rock star (give it all you've got!)
Minute 5: walking lunges (if advanced, add weights)
Minute 6: jumping jacks or jump rope (beginners: quick march)
Minute 7: quick tempo squats this time (45-60 in one minute)
Minute 8: hold plank, then move from forearms to hands, lower and repeat (do not rock through the hips while moving)
Minute 9: speed-walk or run as fast as you can
Minute 10: V-ups*

Be sure to take a few minutes to cool-down and stretch afterwards. Use the following link if you need a guide for stretching: http://www.mayoclinic.com/health/stretching/SM00043&slide=2

❏ Email or text your partner: "I did Day 49's Take Ten 3 times today, and it was ....!"

You only have 22 "Don't just stand there, move!" minutes left to complete today! You can do it! 10+10+10+22 = 52

Should I exercise if I am...

Pregnant or Breastfeeding?
Light to moderately intense exercise is generally safe in pregnancy, but always get clearance from your OB before starting a new exercise program or increasing intensity. I suggest taking on the exercises suggested in the "Take Tens" slowly. Be sure to build in extra time to transition from one minute's exercise to the next, and for cooling down when you are finished. Exercise is generally safe for nursing mothers, but be sure to stay hydrated and eat enough calories so that your milk production does not decline.

Sick?
Typically people eat less when they are sick, and thus stay in caloric balance without exercising on the days they feel especially poor. The general rule for exercise when you don't feel great is if it's "above the neck," you can go ahead with moderately intense exercise. Studies show that regular, moderate exercise can boost your immunity against respiratory infections. Remember that while you are sick, what you eat will make most of the caloric impact for the day, so carefully choose healthy foods that will keep you strong for when you can return to more intense exercise.

Injured?
If you are injured, restrict activity for at least 48 to 72 hours. The PRICE principle should be used in directing your next steps:
P – Protect from further injury
R – Restrict activity (gentle activity may be appropriate)
I – Apply Ice (for 15-20 minutes every 60-90 minutes)
C – Apply Compression
E – Elevate the injured area
For detailed information regarding injuries, visit http://www.acsm.org/docs/brochures/sprains-strains-and-tears.pdf. Pain is your body's way of alerting you to a problem, so if pain continues, consult your medical care provider.

Note: If you are too sick to exercise during your 52 day Countdown, write "sick" across the check-box related to exercise, but do your best to complete the rest of the challenges assigned to that day.

Day 48

- ❑ 64+ ounces of "REAL" water
- ❑ Move for 52 minutes. You are getting great at this!
- ❑ Consume no more than 5 grams of added sugar daily (see label for "sugars") from food or beverages - just for 3 more days!
- ❑ Fill half of your plate at lunch and dinner with non-starchy veggies.

Tracking your food helps you to become more aware of your intake - especially how much sugar you are consuming. So for the next 3 days, log everything you eat or drink on an electronic food tracker such as MyFitnessPal.com (or the app), Supertracker.usda.gov, livestrong.com, or sparkpeople.com. (You can sync up with your partner on My Fitness Pal if desired.)

Food logging, or tracking, is a huge eye-opener! This discipline helps you to pay attention to what you are putting into your mouth, and how much. Then it gives you immediate feedback so you know how to gauge the rest of your day's calories. This process will help you to become more mindful of your eating, and if it keeps you from popping things into your mouth unnecessarily, then I would encourage you to continue keeping records until you have this habit under control.

The electronic tracking system that you use will not consider your medical or weight history when it gives you an estimated calorie range. Please only take the calorie goal provided by generalized programs as a guide. If it seems like too little or too much food for you, or if you adhere to the calorie level suggested and your weight changes unfavorably, consult a registered dietitian for a customized calorie level and meal plan.

- ❑ Every single bite and sip needs to be entered into your food log...just for 3 days. Please do not log your exercise into any of the online tracking programs, and if you have a Fit Bit or something similar, please consider only your food calories. Entering in your exercise will often bump your calories up beyond what you should be consuming (especially while trying to lose weight). Sometimes that might prompt you to eat more than you need at the end of the night to "meet" your day's caloric needs considering your exercise.

Until I entered it into the food tracking app on my phone, I didn't realize that one Otis Spunkmeyer blueberry muffin could take up ALL my breakfast calories all by itself by 7:00 am (400 calories)! And I just bought a whole pack of them from Sam's!

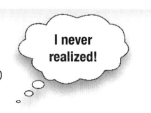
I never realized!

Patrice, 42

Log your food below if you are unable to enter it directly into an online tracking program or app. If you are writing down your intake below, please do transfer this information to an electronic food tracker so you can get immediate feedback. If you find it helps you to jot down your intake on a hard copy, the document below is also in Appendix E for you to make copies for daily use, or download it from my website: bestbodyin52.com.

FOOD LOG DATE:	WHEN AND WHERE?	HUNGER BEFORE AND SATIETY AFTER
BREAKFAST		0 1 2 3 4 5 6 7 8 9 10 Starving Content Stuffed
		0 1 2 3 4 5 6 7 8 9 10 Starving Content Stuffed
SNACK		0 1 2 3 4 5 6 7 8 9 10 Starving Content Stuffed
LUNCH		0 1 2 3 4 5 6 7 8 9 10 Starving Content Stuffed
		0 1 2 3 4 5 6 7 8 9 10 Starving Content Stuffed
SNACK		0 1 2 3 4 5 6 7 8 9 10 Starving Content Stuffed

FOOD LOG DATE:	WHEN AND WHERE?	HUNGER BEFORE AND SATIETY AFTER
DINNER		0 1 2 3 4 5 6 7 8 9 10 Starving · Content · Stuffed 0 1 2 3 4 5 6 7 8 9 10 Starving · Content · Stuffed
NOTES: ❑ I REACHED MY WATER GOAL!		

Day 47

❑ 64+ ounces of "REAL" water

❑ Consume no more than 5 grams of added sugar daily (see label for "sugars") from food or beverages - just for 2 more days!

❑ Fill half of your plate at lunch and dinner with non-starchy veggies.

❑ REST from vigorous exercise today, but make sure you are on your feet being active at least 52 minutes of the day. Also, twice weekly on rest days throughout the Countdown, you will have the opportunity to improve your plank time, not to mention strengthen your abs, back, hips, shoulders, and arms. You will be amazed at the improvement in your core strength over the course of the Countdown if you stay committed to this at least twice a week when assigned.

❑ Time your plank; how long can you hold it with good form before you need to stop? ____minutes and _____seconds

❑ Did you log your food again today? _____ If not, please think through your day and spend a moment logging every bite and sip. If you are unable to enter it directly into an electronic tracking program or app, make a copy of Appendix E to log your food. Remember to transfer this information to an electronic food tracker. Having that feedback right away may help you make better choices as the day goes on.

❑ Look over your log and think about how you did. If I were a little angel peeking over your shoulder, what would I say?

....

....

Did you know that 40-50 years ago the average American slept one or two hours longer per night? Your Best Body in-the-making needs rest to reach its full potential. Studies show that those who stay up very late eat an average of 300-550 calories more since they are awake longer. It's not that calories consumed at night are not burned off efficiently; rather the calorie-dense food choices that are made late at night when you are tired, and often alone, are simply more than your body needs for fuel. They are therefore efficiently saved as body fat.

Which of the following are you more likely to eat after 11 pm? (circle)
- buttered popcorn or raw veggie sticks?
- ice cream or Greek yogurt?
- a bowl of cereal or an apple?
- leftover pizza or a salad?

Therein lies my point! Sometimes the nourishment we need is sleep, not food. Before you get hungry enough for another meal's worth of calories, it is best to turn off the lights (and all your electronic devices) and go to sleep.

❑ Be sure to sleep a *minimum* of 7 hours tonight and every night during the 47 days remaining, and beyond. When you don't get enough sleep, your body secretes a hormone called ghrelin that may increase your appetite and reduce the sensation of fullness you should get after a meal. These changes may promote weight gain and increase your risk of developing chronic disease. A growing body of research suggests that those who sleep six hours or less a night have an increased risk of diabetes, obesity, heart disease, and insulin resistance.

Did you know that alcohol and caffeine intake have been shown to disturb sleep? What do you need to change in your routine in order to prioritize good quality sleep?

....

....

....

Mark an "X" below to show where you think you stand on this continuum:

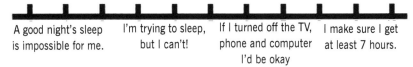

A good night's sleep is impossible for me.   I'm trying to sleep, but I can't!   If I turned off the TV, phone and computer I'd be okay   I make sure I get at least 7 hours.

Getting plenty of sleep will make your other efforts over the course of this Countdown more effective! Another vital piece to making your hard work obvious is choosing lean protein over high fat or heavily processed meats. The evidence won't only be in how your clothes look on you, but also in how your labs look in your medical chart. Even if you are young and your heart health is not a concern on your radar, keep in mind that build-up in the arteries can start before the teen years, and more than half of Americans die of heart disease. Regardless of your age, you want your arteries to be as clean as your hands are before dinner.

Protein is an essential part of your diet, coming mostly from animal products such as fish, meat, eggs, and dairy; protein-fortified bars, shakes, and cereals; and beans and nuts. Protein needs to be part of each meal and snack to help hold you over to the next meal, and also to repair your muscles from the slight healthy damage caused by your workouts.

The amount of protein you need daily depends of course on your "vehicle size and use." Refer to the Pounds and Calories section of the Success Journal if you need a refresher of this analogy. Active people (that's you!) need to aim for about 20 grams of protein or more at each of three daily meals. Snacks should ideally contain protein as well. You'll learn more about snacks on Day 45, but feel free to peek ahead. Below are some tips to keep in mind when it comes to protein:
• Aim for 2-3 servings of fish weekly (2-5 ounces per serving), choosing fish high in omega-3 fatty acids as often as possible (salmon, mackerel, herring, lake trout, sardines and albacore tuna).
• Steer clear of fried fish and fried meats; instead, broil, bake, stew, or grill.
• When choosing poultry, choose white meat most often and remove the skin where the unhealthy saturated fat is found.
• Cheese is a good protein source, but also contributes greatly to most of my clients' fat and calories over the course of the day. Try not to have it more than once a day, and always aim for the reduced-

fat versions (part-skim mozzarella is naturally reduced-fat).

• When choosing red meat, limit it to one serving of lean beef and one serving of lean pork weekly. Go for the "loin" or "round" cuts, and choose "choice" or "select" grades over "prime." Before cooking, trim off as much fat as you can, and after cooking pour off any liquid fat.

• Avoid processed meats such as sausage, bologna, salami and hot dogs. Most of them are high in sodium, preservatives, calories, and saturated fat (the artery-clogging kind of fat). Consider cooking extra portions of lean meat and slicing it thinly to freeze for use on sandwiches as needed.

• One egg is equivalent in protein to one ounce of meat. Egg whites and yolks both contain protein, but the yolks are high in cholesterol. For those with heart disease, the American Heart Association recommends no more than 2 yolks per week.

Lean cuts of meat tend to cost more, so I recommend buying them in bulk when they are on sale, or from a warehouse club such as Sam's or Costco. Remember, you can spend your money on healthy choices now or, perhaps, on medications or surgeries to treat the consequences of poor choices later.

Q: What about vegetarians   FAQ
or those who don't eat meat daily?

A: Vegetarians can typically meet protein needs with milk, Greek yogurt, eggs, cheese, cottage cheese, protein-fortified cereals and bars, beans, nuts, and soy products such as tofu. Vegans have to be especially intentional to get protein needs met. Nuts and beans contain protein, but for a high calorie cost, so I primarily count nuts as fat and beans as starch (see Appendix J for serving sizes).

For example, to get the same amount of protein from almonds that you do from a 160-calorie, 3 1/2 ounce chicken breast (25 g protein), you would need to eat 3/4 cup of almonds at the cost of 715 calories and 65 grams of fat (the total daily fat recommended for a 2000 calorie diet). In average portions, the protein contribution of beans and nuts is low to moderate. They should therefore be combined with other moderate-protein foods (such as whole wheat noodles) over the course of the day to cumulatively meet protein needs. Anyone avoiding major food groups should take a daily multivitamin/multimineral supplement. Those who do not eat meat regularly need a vitamin B12 supplement orally or by way of injection.

Garlic Pork Loin

Serves 10

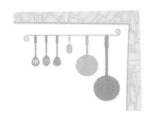

1 boneless pork loin (about 3 pounds)
3 large cloves garlic, minced
Cracked pepper, to taste

1. Set the pork on a cutting board. Make tiny slits all over the meat on both sides and insert the garlic, pushing it into the meat.
2. Sprinkle with cracked pepper and rub it over both sides of the loin.
3. Refrigerate for a couple hours or for as long as overnight.
4. Turn on the broiler. Set the pork in a roasting pan covered with foil.
5. Broil for 10 minutes on each side, or until golden.
6. Turn the oven down to 400 degrees. Continue roasting for 30-40 minutes or until the center of the pork registers 140 degrees on a meat thermometer for pink meat or 150 degrees for well-done meat.
7. After removing it from the oven, flip over the meat and loosely wrap it in foil, letting it sit for 5 minutes. The temperature will rise about 5 degrees.
8. Slice the loin thinly and serve at once.
Freeze extras for use as sandwich meat in the place of processed deli meat.

Nutrient Breakdown (in 3-1/2 ounces.): Calories 152, Fat 5 g, (2 g sat fat), Sodium 41 mg, Carbohydrate 0 g, Fiber 0 g, Protein 24 g

Day 46

❏ 64+ ounces of "REAL" water
❏ Move for 52 minutes
❏ Consume no more than 5
grams of added sugar daily (see label for "sugars") from food or beverages - just for this last day! If desired, starting tomorrow you can double your added sugar grams, but if you find your sugar cravings increase as your sugar intake increases, then stick with just 5 grams.
❏ Fill half of your plate at lunch and dinner with non-starchy veggies.

Some people eat several small meals or "graze" all day, and some people eat just one big meal a day. I have seen both of these cause trouble. Grazers often don't get a good balance, as they usually do not get enough protein or vegetables. Research shows those that eat just once a day are more likely to be overweight or obese.

I recommend eating 4-5 times daily: breakfast, lunch, and dinner, plus a mid-afternoon "Strong Snack" combining the three food types in the upcoming chart. If you have long, active days, you may need to add another "Strong Snack" mid-morning. You will see shortly that it is more like a small meal than a snack.

Aim to eat about the same number of calories each time you eat - 4 (or 5) times a day - wrapping up with dinner. This keeps your blood sugar and hunger levels balanced so that you do not end up overeating or binging when you get too hungry. Eating balanced meals in regular intervals also keeps your metabolism from getting sluggish. Using My Fitness Pal or a similar electronic tracking program/app to help you balance out your calories throughout the day is ideal.

It works!

"I have been eating the same number of calories for breakfast, lunch, "Strong Snack" and dinner like you taught me, and I've maintained my weight for two years now! It works perfectly for me!"

Ciara, 37

❑   Log your food today. Look over your food records from the past 3 days and choose the most typical day to complete the blanks below. Fill in the numbers to learn what your balance of calories looks like:

First 4 hours of your day:	_____calories
Second 4 hours of your day:	_____calories
Third 4-hour block of your day:	_____calories
Fourth 4-hour block of your day:	_____calories
Last hours of your day, if applicable:	_____calories

The purpose of this is not to get you caught up in counting calories, as the Countdown focuses more on being aware of them than running a tally. Fueling in balanced increments from the start of the day, when you likely need the energy most, helps to prevent the overeating that often results from waiting to eat until you "have time" later in the day. The goal of this particular assignment is to emphasize the importance of balancing your intake over the course of your wakeful hours. That means at first you will have to do some investigating, which includes assessing your day's calorie balance.

Your body will operate best when good nutrition is available to your cells all day long. You will also be less likely to overeat later in the day. Did you eat about the same number of calories over each of the 4-hour segments of your day?.................. If not, what do you need to adjust in order to even things out a little?

....

....

"Strong Snacks"

Choose one from each category below (the amount from the third column depends on your activity level). This combination typically ensures a minimum of 5 grams of protein and 3 grams of fiber, both of which help to hold you over gracefully until your final meal. Choosing one item from each column will be about a 200-300 calorie snack. If you are especially active, you may need to add a second fat and a grain.

DAIRY OR ALTERNATIVE	FRUIT (LOOK FOR FIBER AND COLOR VARIETY!)	HEALTHY FAT (1 FAT SERVING= 50 CALORIES)
1 cup milk (fat free or 1%), or 1 cup soy milk, rice milk or almond milk	1/2 banana or any other fruit (see portion sizes in Appendix J)	pecans or walnuts: 4 halves (50 calories) or 8 halves (100 calories)
6-8 ounces of yogurt (go for Greek)	3/4 cup raspberries or any other berries	sunflower seeds (1 tbsp = 50 calories)
1/4 cup Fat Free or 1% cottage cheese	1 orange, or any other tennis-ball sized fruit	large olives - 8 black, 10 green (stuffed)
string cheese piece	1 medium apple, sliced	1-1/2 tsp peanut butter
milk with cereal noted to the right:	occasional cereal substitute: look for >3 grams of protein and >2 g fiber in a 15 gram carb portion (see label)	10 peanuts or 16 pistachios (50 calories) almonds or cashews 6 (50) or 12 (100)
1.5 ounce of reduced fat cheese	occasional substitute: 15 grams carb portion of whole grain crackers	2 tablespoons avocado (1/5th of an avocado)

Q: What if I am not hungry for a "Strong Snack?"

A: If you can go from noon to the typical 6:30-7:00 pm dinner with no need for a snack, I would suggest you "drive your car around more often" to use up your "fuel." (Look back to the Pounds and Calories section of the Success Journal for details). Or, if you are active, but still are not hungry during the day, consider the following:
• you could be eating too heavy a lunch for your caloric expenditure, or having sugar between meals from drinks or candy that holds you over
• perhaps a medication you are on, or stress, may suppress your appetite
• your metabolism may be sluggish due to low caloric intake over time, yo-yo dieting, or use of appetite suppressants or other medications that have this side effect
• you might be eating an early enough dinner that you simply do not need a snack (but watch out for evening hunger)
Try not to skip meals or go more than 5 hours without eating a meal or "Strong Snack."

Just a heads up: you'll need to be ready in the morning to take pictures of tomorrow's breakfast.

Log your food on a copy of Appendix E today if you are unable to enter it into an online tracking program or app until later.

Did you transfer this information to an electronic food tracker?

....

It may have been a challenging week, but you made it through! If you can do the first week, you can surely finish the 52 days strong! Be aware that when something throws off your routine, like illness, work/school schedule changes, or going out of town, it's typical to get off track. Don't let a bump in the road cause you to give up! You can pick up on the same day, or back up a few days, but don't quit before you reach Your Best Body! What are you going to do if you happen to get off track for a day or two of the Countdown?

....

....

60

Day 45

Okay, that was the toughest week of the Countdown! You should be proud of yourself! You have dug deep to lay the foundation for your success. Picture yourself safely within the fortress you are building that will protect your health. Every day until you have reached Your Best Body goals, you will add to the five key building blocks to

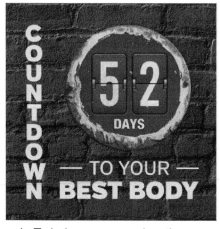

which you have just been introduced. To help you remember these foundational basics to reaching Your Best Body, think "Countdown 5, 4, 3, 2, 1."

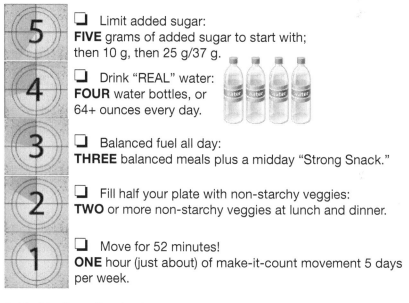

❑ Limit added sugar:
FIVE grams of added sugar to start with; then 10 g, then 25 g/37 g.

❑ Drink "REAL" water:
FOUR water bottles, or 64+ ounces every day.

❑ Balanced fuel all day:
THREE balanced meals plus a midday "Strong Snack."

❑ Fill half your plate with non-starchy veggies:
TWO or more non-starchy veggies at lunch and dinner.

❑ Move for 52 minutes!
ONE hour (just about) of make-it-count movement 5 days per week.

Added to these five fundamentals, the challenges and tips for each day of the Countdown will be like the mortar that keeps you building on the foundation you have established.

❑ Starting today, allow a maximum of 10 grams of added sugar daily from foods and beverages - just for these next 7 days. It's much easier than 5 grams, but it still adds up quickly. For example, in just one packet of maple and brown sugar flavored oatmeal, there are 12 grams of added sugar! After this week, we will finish out the rest of the Countdown at a maximum of 25 grams of added sugar or less for women, and 37 for men.

Q: Which kind of milk should I use?

A: There are several types of milk, all of which have different nutritional profiles and varying benefits. I believe they should be varied, just as all your foods should be. For example, use dairy products for cheese and yogurt, use plain soy milk or cow's milk with breakfast for more protein to hold you through the morning, and use almond milk when you need the calories as low as possible and have already met your protein needs for that segment of the day, like when having a treat such as the Coffee and Cream Shake.

❑ Eat breakfast within about 45 minutes of waking up every day. Eating breakfast jump-starts your engine and gets you fueled and alert for an active day! It's also when most people get the bulk of their fiber needs met for the day. If you are already starting the day strong, then it's time for a breakfast check-up.

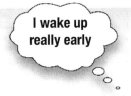
I wake up really early

I wake up really early for work and just can't stomach eating breakfast yet, so I eat a piece of fruit and then have the rest of my breakfast when I get to work.

Sabrina, 29

❑ Open your pantry and get out a variety of three items that have labels, and three from your refrigerator as well. To assess your breakfast and to complete upcoming days of the Countdown, you'll need to get acquainted with your food labels.
 1) Locate the Nutrition Facts Panel
 2) Locate Serving Size and Calories
 3) Locate Total Fat, Saturated Fat and Trans Fat (the latter two are the ones that damage your heart)

4) Locate Total Carbohydrate, Dietary Fiber, and Sugars
5) Locate Protein
6) Locate the Ingredient List

❑ Locate and review those 6 important parts of a label on each packaged item that you eat all day. If that seems laborious, maybe it will prompt you to eat more fresh, whole foods today that don't come out of a package.

The Best Body Breakfast:

❑ 10 grams fiber (minimum) from 1-3 grain servings (depending on your fuel needs and activity level), and 1 fruit serving (see Appendix J for serving sizes of common foods, and refer to the table on Day 38 for a list of common foods containing fiber).

❑ 15-30 grams of protein (from all of the food groups combined)

❑ 300-500 mg calcium (typically found in 1 dairy serving noted below):

- skim or 1% milk or yogurt (1 cup)
- reduced fat cheese (1.5 ounces)
- low fat cottage cheese (1/4 cup)
- a dairy alternative fortified with calcium such as soy milk, rice-milk, almond milk, or orange juice (see product label for calcium quantity)
- or a 300-500 mg supplement

❑ 5-15 grams of fat, ideally from a small serving of nuts
(Refer to the serving sizes of various fats in Appendix J. The healthy fats are listed toward the top of the column for fats, and the those most likely to damage your heart are listed toward the bottom. Though fat should be part of every meal, all fats should be portion-controlled due to their caloric density. For detailed serving sizes for specific nuts, see the table on page 59).

❑ Starting with your "Best Body Breakfast," take a picture of each of today's 3 meals and your "Strong Snack," and email or text them to your partner.

If you just cannot manage to eat breakfast in the first hour of your day, carefully plan so that your morning mini-meals add up to meet my Best Breakfast guidelines over the first 3-4 hours of your day.

Day 44

5 ❏ Limit added sugar:
FIVE grams of added sugar to start with;
then 10 g, then 25 g/37 g.

4 ❏ Drink "REAL" water:
FOUR water bottles, or
64+ ounces every day.

3 ❏ Balanced fuel all day:
THREE balanced meals plus a midday "Strong Snack."

2 ❏ Fill half your plate with non-starchy veggies:
TWO or more non-starchy veggies at lunch and dinner.

1 ❏ Move for 52 minutes!
ONE hour (just about) of make-it-count movement 5
days per week..

❏ Allow a maximum of 10 grams of added sugar daily - just for
these next 6 days. That's about 2 teaspoons of added sugar per day.
Remember added sugar is not just table sugar. Consider the following
as added sugars as well: evaporated cane juice, dextrose, any corn
syrup, brown sugar, molasses, and honey.

❏ Rest today, but time your plank; how long can you hold it with good
form before you need to stop? ....minutes and ....seconds

❏ Barrier Buster! Write down 10 barriers or excuses that could get in
your way of success. You must be aware of temptations and dangers
that you simply cannot allow in your path. However, being aware is only
half of the battle, so next write out 10 corresponding solutions.

BARRIER	BARRIER BUSTER
allowing myself to get too hungry only to over-eat later	eat 4 times daily (or 5) - that's 3 meals plus a "Strong Snack" daily with protein, fiber and healthy fat
buying snacks for the kids' sports teams	buy only enough for the kids; store on the top shelf in a container labeled "Kids only"
making excuses for myself	own my choices, accept the consequences, and press on
eating popcorn at the movies	eat healthy popcorn before going; bring exact change for the movie (no cards or extra cash)
waiting to exercise "later"	bring exercise wear when leaving home for the day; exercise before returning home
giving up if I gain a pound or eat poorly	if I get off track or gain a pound, I will start the week afresh and not give up
1.	
2.	
3.	
4.	
5.	
6.	
7.	
8.	
9.	
10.	

Q: What can I have to satisfy my sweet tooth?   Robin, 36

A: The Countdown started you at no more than 5 grams of added sugar and this week you are allotted 10 grams. I recommend a maximum of 25 grams of added sugar daily as a long term lifestyle change for women, and 37 grams for men. The sweet tooth satisfiers I will suggest stay under that limit, but since I'm urging you to do this for the long haul, I know there will be exceptions like your Birthday or Valentines Day. Your body can adjust to those rare exceptions, just be careful that they don't sneakily become the norm. Try to keep desserts to a 100 calorie maximum, and for most desserts that means bumping about one fat serving and one grain/starch serving from your day. Some of my favorites are below. If you need to sweeten the yogurt, you can use Stevia or Splenda.

Sweet-Tooth Satisfiers

CREAMY:
• add about 60 Ghirardelli mini semi-sweet chocolate baking chips (that's about 2 tablespoons - just 35 calories and 4 grams of added sugar) to unsweetened plain Greek yogurt with 3/4 cup of chopped strawberries
CRUNCHY:
• if it's a cookie you are after, think "small is better than not at all" and know you'll have to bump a grain/starch serving, plus a fat serving to make room in your day for 2 Oreos, for example
HOT:
• 1 packet of Swiss Miss 25 calorie hot chocolate, plus 2 tablespoons mini-marshmallows (totaling 45 calories, 4 g added sugar)
COLD:
• frozen blueberries (3/4 cup = 1 fruit serving, 0 g added sugar)
• "Coffee and Cream Shake"

Coffee and Cream Shake

Serves 1

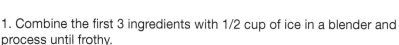

1/4 cup Edy's Slow Churned French Silk Ice Cream
3 ounces black coffee, chilled
3 ounces unsweetened almond milk
cinnamon to taste

1. Combine the first 3 ingredients with 1/2 cup of ice in a blender and process until frothy.
2. Sprinkle with cinnamon and serve immediately.

Nutrient Breakdown: Calories 78, Fat 5 g, Carb 11 g, Fiber 0 g, Protein 3 g, Sodium 60 g, Sugars 8 g (about 6 g of which is added sugar)

If purchasing the ingredients for these treats and having them on hand will cause you to be tempted to overdo it, what should you do?

....

Day 43

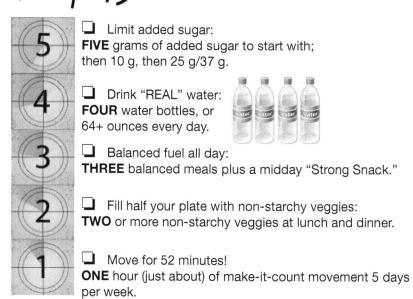

❏ Limit added sugar:
FIVE grams of added sugar to start with; then 10 g, then 25 g/37 g.

❏ Drink "REAL" water:
FOUR water bottles, or 64+ ounces every day.

❏ Balanced fuel all day:
THREE balanced meals plus a midday "Strong Snack."

❏ Fill half your plate with non-starchy veggies:
TWO or more non-starchy veggies at lunch and dinner.

❏ Move for 52 minutes!
ONE hour (just about) of make-it-count movement 5 days per week.

❏ Allow a maximum of 10 grams of added sugar daily - just for 5 more days.

To improve metabolism, definition, strength, muscle mass, and bone mass, not to mention burn extra calories around the clock, the ideal is to work all major muscle groups 2 to 3 times per week. Are you currently doing that weekly?............ If not, try to do so. You can typically see initial results and gain strength in just 4-6 weeks of consistency! But, if you just "dabble" in it, you may instead be immobilized by soreness after each infrequent time you work those muscles.

This is worth committing to, especially if you already exercise regularly, but have never been consistent with strength or resistance training. If you have been faithfully doing strength exercises, keep in mind that you must continually challenge the muscles. You can't just do the same exercises with the same resistance and expect ongoing progress. I tell my Monday morning strength class that I need a doctor's excuse if they are going to lift light weights (unless they are still beginners...in that case I give them four Mondays). They know I'm joking, but they get the message that I want them to make it worth their while.

It may seem intimidating at first, but strength training just might be what changes the look of your body the most!

❏ Incorporate strength/resistance training into your workouts at least 1 time weekly. The "Take Ten" you recently did is a great start. Strength/resistance classes or videos are the perfect way to get all major muscle groups worked in one hour. Or, consider a personal trainer to get you acquainted if you are new to it, or to push you to the next level if you are not a beginner.

❏ If you are already consistent with strength training, brainstorm how can you vary your exercises to challenge yourself. Check one that you will try this week:

- ○ increase your weight/resistance, or repetitions
- ○ try a class format you haven't tried before
- ○ change from machines to free weights or vice versa
- ○ use body-weight exercises (for example, push-ups and side planks)
- ○ other: ....

Q: I've been doing these tough "Take Tens" every other day and sometimes I feel nauseous during exercise. What should I do?

A: If you feel sick, most likely you just need to take it down a notch in terms of intensity and be sure to transition slowly from one thing to the next, especially if it involves getting on the floor from a standing position or vice versa. If you need to pull back and take a break, dial your intensity down gradually rather than just stopping short. It is best to keep moving slowly so that blood does not pool in your extremities causing you to get dizzy and possibly faint. Typically this improves as you become more fit. Also, it is possible that you ate too close to your workout or that you are too hungry. Think back to the last time you ate and change the timing to make it work for you.

Have you logged your weight for the week on Appendix C's graph? .... If you were planning to lose weight this week, how do you feel about your progress so far?

....
....

Day 42

❏ Limit added sugar: **FIVE** grams of added sugar to start with; then 10 g, then 25 g/37 g.

❏ Drink "REAL" water: **FOUR** water bottles, or 64+ ounces every day.

❏ Balanced fuel all day: **THREE** balanced meals plus a midday "Strong Snack."

69

❏ Fill half your plate with non-starchy veggies:
TWO or more non-starchy veggies at lunch and dinner.

❏ Move for 52 minutes!
ONE hour (just about) of make-it-count movement 5 days per week.

❏ Allow a maximum of 10 grams of added sugar daily - just for 4 more days.

Congratulations! You've made it 10 days already! Let's see how your changes are beginning to impact your life.

✳ Have you been drinking water consistently every day?....................
If you weren't before, has it helped you:
    ❏ feel more full?
    ❏ become more "regular?"
    ❏ have fewer headaches?
    ❏ feel less sluggish?

✳ Have you been moving for 52 minutes a day, 5 days a week (at least half of it being intense)?...............
Are you:
    ❏ feeling more energetic?
    ❏ sleeping better?
    ❏ feeling stronger?
    ❏ becoming more "regular?"
    ❏ less stressed?

If you were already doing this, what have you changed in order to reach Your Best Body?

....
....

✳ When exercising, are you working at a 6.5 - 9 intensity level (on a scale of 1-10) at least half of the 52 minutes?...........................

✳ How difficult for you has it been to cut back on added sugar?

❏ extremely difficult   ❏ not too bad
❏ pretty tough   ❏ no biggie

✳ List some foods that have more added sugar than you realized:

....

....

✳ Could eating sugar/sweets be contributing to poor health, increased disease risk, or extra pounds for you? Explain:

....

....

✳ Do you think you can maintain 25 grams of added sugar for women/37 grams for men, as your added sugar maximum all the way through the Countdown? ....If not, why not?

....

....

✳ Has it made a difference to keep tempting foods out of your reach, and to minimize those discouragers? Explain.

....

....

✳ Do you feel: (circle)   more in control?   empowered?

✳ What about progress in the area of your weight? Your thoughts?

....

✳ Are you in the habit of filling your plate half full of non-starchy veggies? .... If not, this is critical! What can you do to ensure this happens? (check)

     ❏ I need to try some different veggies.
     ❏ I need to try new ways to prepare veggies I don't typically like.
     ❏ I will add more veggies to my soups and hot dishes.
     ❏ I will plan to keep raw, ready-to-eat veggies on hand.
     ❏ I need to buy pre-chopped salads and ready-to-eat vegetables to make eating them more convenient.
     ❏ I will double the amount of veggies I cook so there are always some ready to add to my next meal.
     ❏ Other: ....

✳ Did the "Take Ten" encourage you to consider ways to get brief workouts in when you don't have a lot of time?...........................

✳ When could you do this again this week (or even something similar like go for a brisk walk/jog for 10-15 minutes before showering)?
....

✳ Has tracking your food made a difference for you? If so, how?
....
....

✳ When you eat a breakfast that follows my Best Body Breakfast guidelines, have you noticed any of the following?
- ❏ improved energy level
- ❏ a boost in concentration
- ❏ better satiety
- ❏ more "regular"
- ❏ better fueled for workouts
- ❏ Other:...

✳ Has removing any of those barriers you listed made a difference yet? Explain:
....
....

✳ Please go back to Day 44 now and highlight the "Barrier Busters" you still need to work on.
- ❏ Check here when you have done so.

✳ What is your plan for regularly incorporating strength training? Which days of the week, how, and where?
....
....

✳ Flip back through your Success Journal. Have you marked off most of the daily check-boxes so far on this journey to Your Best Body? ....

✳ Place an "X" on the following continuum to indicate your commitment level to finishing this Countdown with a Success Journal full of check-boxes and responses on every line.

| | | | | | | | | |
Not likely   I think I can.   Yes! I can do it!

✳ Three things I have done well:

1...

2...

3...

✳ Based on this assessment of my progress, three things I'm going to focus on starting today are:

1...

2...

3...

"I long to accomplish a great and noble task, but it is my chief duty to accomplish small tasks as if they were great and noble."

Helen Keller

Day 41

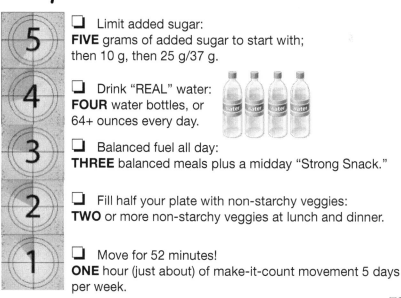

❏ Limit added sugar:
FIVE grams of added sugar to start with; then 10 g, then 25 g/37 g.

❏ Drink "REAL" water:
FOUR water bottles, or 64+ ounces every day.

❏ Balanced fuel all day:
THREE balanced meals plus a midday "Strong Snack."

❏ Fill half your plate with non-starchy veggies:
TWO or more non-starchy veggies at lunch and dinner.

❏ Move for 52 minutes!
ONE hour (just about) of make-it-count movement 5 days per week.

❏ Allow a maximum of 10 grams of added sugar daily - just for 3 more days.

❏ Strive to get fruits and veggies in today from each color in the rainbow. The deeper and brighter their colors, often the more power-packed the vegetables and fruits are. To prioritize them, bump chips and snack-foods for veggies, and replace desserts with fruits. Below are some suggestions; the **produce in bold** rates the highest in nutrients and fiber.

If you are watching your weight, keep in mind that the veggies with the * are considered starches (or legumes), which are 3 times as calorie-dense as the non-starchy veggies. Remember, they need to share space with your grains on just a quarter of your plate. Those with the ** are considered healthy fats and they are about 5 times as calorie-dense as the non-starchy vegetables listed. They should take up just about a thumb-print of space on your plate. Refer to Appendix J for the appropriate serving sizes for the fats listed.

Red:
strawberries, tomatoes, tomato sauce, **watermelon, red bell pepper,** cherries, beets, raspberries, apples, **grapefruit, radishes**

Orange:
dried apricots (or fresh), **sweet potato*, orange,** peach, **carrots,** nectarine, **pumpkin, grapefruit, cantaloupe,** orange bell pepper, tangerine, **butternut squash**

Yellow:
banana, squash (lots of types!), **mango,** yellow bell pepper, pineapple, lemon, pear, corn*, garlic, onions, cauliflower (well, yellow-ish)

Green:
broccoli, green grapes, spinach, **kiwi,** celery, honeydew melon, lettuce, lime, starfruit, okra, **various leafy greens,** cucumbers, **green bell pepper, brussels sprouts, peas*,** snow peas, asparagus, zucchini, artichoke, lima beans*, green beans, cabbage/coleslaw, olives**, avocado**

Blue/Violet:
blueberries, eggplant, plums, blackberries, figs, **red cabbage, radicchio,** red onions

74

The Environmental Working Group puts out an annual "Dirty Dozen" list in order to help consumers decide which fruits and vegetables are worth spending extra dollars on based on detected pesticide residue levels. Though they cost a little more, when possible, try to choose organic produce for the "Dirty Dozen:"

Apples	Nectarines (imported)
Celery	Peaches
Cherry tomatoes	Potatoes
Cucumbers	Spinach
Grapes	Strawberries
Hot peppers	Sweet bell peppers

Can you recall three reasons to prioritize vegetables so that they fill up about half of your plate twice a day?

1...

2...

3...

Day 40

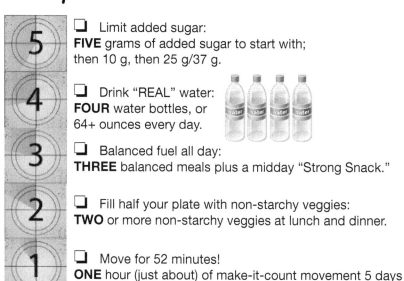

❏ Limit added sugar:
FIVE grams of added sugar to start with; then 10 g, then 25 g/37 g.

❏ Drink "REAL" water:
FOUR water bottles, or 64+ ounces every day.

❏ Balanced fuel all day:
THREE balanced meals plus a midday "Strong Snack."

❏ Fill half your plate with non-starchy veggies:
TWO or more non-starchy veggies at lunch and dinner.

❏ Move for 52 minutes!
ONE hour (just about) of make-it-count movement 5 days per week.

❑ Allow a maximum of 10 grams of added sugar daily - just for 2 more days.

❑ Rest today, but time your plank; how long can you hold it with good form before you need to stop? ....minutes and .... seconds.

❑ Did you get at least 7 hours of sleep or more per night on average these past 7 days? ....

❑ Trade out refined grains for whole grains today: they increase your fiber intake, boost your antioxidants and promote satiety. Can you make more than half of your daily grains whole grains for the next 40 days? Even better - can you aim to avoid refined grains?

Place an "X" on the continuum below to indicate how likely you are to avoid refined grains for the next 40 days?

| ▮ | ▮ | ▮ | ▮ | ▮ | ▮ | ▮ | ▮ | ▮ |

It's not likely.   I can make half my grains whole.   Only whole grains for me!

How do you know if it is a whole grain? It can be tricky. If the package says 100% whole grain or 100% whole wheat, then it does not contain any refined flour and the product is actually a whole grain product. Look at the first ingredient on your grain label. Whole grains have the word "whole" or say "100%" before the type of grain. Sometimes the next ingredient is a refined flour, so watch out for that and for the following terms which may cause you to think it's a whole grain when it's not: whole grain white, multigrain, 12-grain, good source of whole grain, or made with whole grain. These are simply stating that a whole grain or multiple refined grains were part of the recipe.

Work toward phasing out the refined grains in your home. They don't have the holding power and fiber of the whole-grain options, nor the disease-fighting potential. It can be tough to find whole grains when you're dining out, but you may realize you manage your weight (and your wallet) better when eating out less anyway.

❑ Head over to your pantry and move the refined grains (refer to the following table) to the back of the top shelf, and move the whole grains to front and center, as the better choice.

WHOLE GRAINS	REFINED GRAINS
Steel cut oats and rolled oats	Grits
Whole-grain crackers like Wasa, RyKrisp, Kavli, and Ryvita, Triscuits and Wheat Thins	Ritz, Club or Saltine type crackers
Brown rice or wild rice	White rice
Whole wheat noodles, barley, and quinoa	White (regular) noodles
100% whole grain bread (Pepperidge Farm Stoneground 100% Whole Wheat or Arnold Bakery Light 100% Whole Wheat), whole wheat pita, or Flat Out	White bread, white pitas, tortillas, rolls, pizza dough, biscuits, cookies, pop tarts, sugary breakfast bars
Cheerios, All-bran, whole wheat flake cereals	Any cereals that don't have only whole grains listed, starting with the first ingredient

FAQ

Q: What do you think about going gluten free?

A: There are certainly medical reasons for avoiding gluten, the protein in wheat, barley, and rye (and found in cross-contaminated oats). People who have struggled with various undiagnosed challenges have found much relief when making this change. I have found that many people who feel better on a gluten free diet may feel just as good, without the challenge of going gluten-free, if they:

1) trade out their refined grains for whole grains, choosing products with short ingredient lists and less preservatives

2) vary their grains/starches over the course of the day (intentionally eat grains besides wheat)

3) make sure grain servings fit only on a quarter of their plate, or in the case of bread, limit it to two typical slices on their plate

For example, if I ate a fast food biscuit for breakfast, a sub for lunch with a cookie, and a pile of spaghetti at home for dinner with a side of Italian bread, I'd feel badly and gain weight, too. The research is consistent that going gluten free does not cause weight loss overall, but it just might for you if it prompts you to avoid the calorie-dense foods you were overeating. I suggest trying the three tips I listed above first, as gluten free diets can be expensive and lead to nutritional deficiencies and constipation.

Perfectly Filling Quinoa Lettuce Wraps

Serves 4

Note: these are gluten free, wheat free and egg free

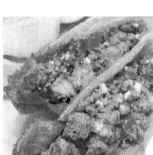

1/2 cup quinoa
1 cup water
2 medium tomatoes
2 cups fresh spinach
1/2 cup green onion, chopped
1 avocado
3 ounces feta cheese
garlic powder, salt, and black pepper (or sparingly use a pre-mixed blend, such as Cavender's Greek Seasoning)
grilled chicken, 8 ounces cooked
romaine lettuce leaves (for boats)

1. Prepare the quinoa by placing 1 cup water on the stove to boil. When the water is boiling, add quinoa, cover and turn down to simmer for 15 minutes, or until the water has been absorbed.
2. Cool in a shallow baking dish in the refrigerator while chopping veggies into small chunks and placing them in a large bowl.
3. Add chilled quinoa to vegetables and toss.
4. Sprinkle with 3 ounces crumbled feta cheese, adding garlic powder, salt and cracked pepper to taste (or mix). Add chunks of grilled chicken.
5. Scoop into romaine lettuce leaves to make lettuce wraps.

Nutrient Breakdown: Calories 359, Fat 12 g, (4 g Sat. Fat), Sodium 398 mg, Carbohydrate 22 g, Fiber 6 g, Protein 32 g

Day 39

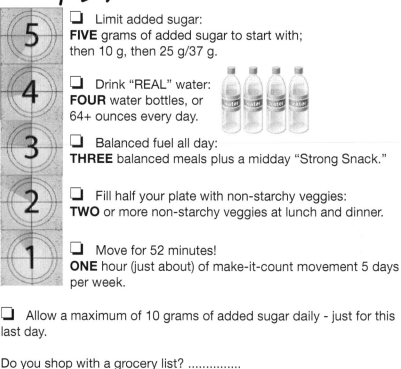

❑ Limit added sugar:
FIVE grams of added sugar to start with; then 10 g, then 25 g/37 g.

❑ Drink "REAL" water:
FOUR water bottles, or 64+ ounces every day.

❑ Balanced fuel all day:
THREE balanced meals plus a midday "Strong Snack."

❑ Fill half your plate with non-starchy veggies:
TWO or more non-starchy veggies at lunch and dinner.

❑ Move for 52 minutes!
ONE hour (just about) of make-it-count movement 5 days per week.

❑ Allow a maximum of 10 grams of added sugar daily - just for this last day.

Do you shop with a grocery list? ....
Is the list based on a menu you planned out ahead of time? ....

> **This is how we shop.**
>
> To make the most of our grocery budget, our family shops as infrequently as possible, planning meals around what is most perishable. We only buy meat on sale or in bulk, limit pricey cereals, and buy just one snack item like crackers per week, otherwise making popcorn on the stove. Our remaining grocery dollars are spent on the healthy basics along the perimeter of the grocery store.
>
> Stephanie, 32

I suggest a shopping trip just once a week, and then if needed, a quick mid-week run to a farmer's market (when that is an option) for produce only. The more often people find themselves in the grocery store, the more likely they are to buy things they don't need or shouldn't eat (think end-caps with sales on candy and chips). Not to mention, that extra 30 minutes in the store may be more wisely spent packing tomorrow's lunch, cooking, or exercising, and the extra dollars on active fun!

Tips for a smart trip to the supermarket:
   • Eat a meal or "Strong Snack" before shopping. Shopping on an empty stomach may lead to indulgent purchases.
   • Make out your meal plan and grocery list before going to the store, and try your best to only buy items off the list when at the store.
   • Stick to the perimeter of the store where most of the whole foods can be found. Avoid going up and down each aisle.
   • Only buy sale items or use coupons if those foods are part of your healthy meal plan. Don't let a sale draw you in to buying something you know is not going to lead to Your Best Body.

❏   Review the Kitchen Clean-Up on page 14. Is your kitchen in better shape now that you have been doing the Countdown for two weeks? .... If not, what still needs to change?

....

....

❏   With the Kitchen Clean-Up in mind, create a list of weekly healthy grocery must-haves using the following Best Body Shopping List. Consider making copies to keep in your kitchen.

To get my recipes and coordinating meal plans, and my brand-specific grocery list, check out "INDESTRUCTIBLE" on my website. The purpose of this web-based accountability is to provide fresh tools and support that keep you from slipping backwards. The website also offers opportunities to share in the journey with others who have committed not to go back to their less-than-Best Bodies, and to have weekly professional support.

bestbodyin52.com

A copy of the following Shopping List template can be found in Appendix F for your convenience.

Appendix F

My BEST BODY Shopping List (think perimeter!)

Fresh produce (did you get all colors of the rainbow?)

_____   _____
_____   _____
_____   _____
_____   _____

Lean meats (fish, poultry & round/loin cuts of pork/beef or tofu)

_____   _____
_____   _____
_____   _____
_____   _____

Whole grains, cereals and beans

_____   _____
_____   _____
_____   _____
_____   _____

Low sodium canned goods and dried fruits

_____   _____
_____   _____

Dairy, eggs, and frozen foods

_____   _____
_____   _____
_____   _____
_____   _____

Day 38

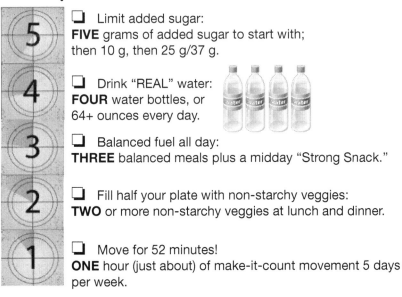

❏ Limit added sugar:
FIVE grams of added sugar to start with; then 10 g, then 25 g/37 g.

❏ Drink "REAL" water:
FOUR water bottles, or 64+ ounces every day.

❏ Balanced fuel all day:
THREE balanced meals plus a midday "Strong Snack."

❏ Fill half your plate with non-starchy veggies:
TWO or more non-starchy veggies at lunch and dinner.

❏ Move for 52 minutes!
ONE hour (just about) of make-it-count movement 5 days per week.

❏ Starting today, and through the rest of the Countdown, allow a maximum of 25 grams of added sugar for women (that's about 100 calories) and 37 grams for men (about 150 calories). This recommendation of the American Heart Association amounts to 6 teaspoons per day of added sugar for women and 9 for men.

Can you stay below the suggested maximum for added sugar for the next 38 days? .... Give it a try! If you choose not to, know that your progress towards reaching Your Best Body will most likely be slower than otherwise.

| I feel like I must have sugar. | This is pretty tough for me. | I have seen enough benefits to stick with this. |

Have you heard of "clean eating?"

I define *"clean eating"* as eating where:

• you don't have to *clean* your hands on four napkins after dinner (think fried chicken)

• you don't have to *clean* wrappers from your counter, table, car or couch after a snack (insert crinkly snack bag sound here)

I think I must be addicted to sugar. I cannot seem to control myself unless I totally stop having it. I almost avoided this Countdown because I didn't think I could make it through that first week with so little sugar. At first it was really hard to break the habit, but after going without it for a couple weeks, it hardly tempts me anymore and I feel so much better!

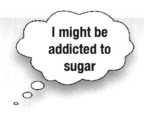

Anonymous, 23

• you don't have to *clean* the grease-based lip-gloss off your lips between bites (think lo-mien)

• you do have to *clean* out your fridge if you go out of town, because most of the food is perishable

• you don't have to *clean* your pizza - that is, you don't have to use your napkin to sop up the fat that puddles on the top (ewww!)

• no need to *clean* salt granules off your table or worry about how much sodium is in everything...because so few of your foods are packaged or canned or cured that the small amount of sodium you are getting from the REAL food you are eating is no big deal (hint: if it has a flavoring packet, or is pre-seasoned, it is likely very high in sodium)

• it won't be as tough to *clean* your frying pan because the lean meats you are using won't leave a saturated mess in the pan

• your body "takes out the trash" every day because your daily fiber-filled foods, your 64+ ounces of "REAL" water, and your exercise are "*cleaning* things out" (need I be more specific?)

• you don't have to take meds to *clean* the buildup out of your arteries, because your food sources containing soluble fiber prevent your digestive system from absorbing cholesterol (read on for a list of fiber-containing foods)

So, today's "clean eating" challenges:

❑ Don't eat any fried or greasy food (remember chips are fried foods, too). Do your best to not eat fried foods for the remainder of the Countdown and beyond.

❑ Clean out your pantry and fridge, removing anything referred to above that you know will hinder your success in reaching Your Best Body. What did you remove?

....

....

❏ Make sure you get 25-35 grams of fiber today and every day. If you typically are nowhere close to that, then inch it up slowly so you don't end up with tummy trouble.

❏ Refer to the food log you did previously to see what you have averaged in fiber grams: ....

Fiber comes mostly from fruits, vegetables, whole grains, beans and nuts. According to the American Heart Association, soluble fiber helps to lower cholesterol and is associated with a decreased risk of cardiovascular disease. I suggest aiming for one serving of soluble fiber-rich foods (denoted on the following chart with *) with each meal. That means that most days of the week, you will need to plan beans into your meals.

FOOD	SERVING SIZE	FIBER (GRAMS)
pear with skin*	1 medium	5.5 grams
apple with skin*	1 medium	4.4 grams
strawberries*	3/4 cup	3.0 grams
orange*	1 medium	3.1 grams
whole wheat pasta	1/2 cup	3.2 grams
barley, cooked*	1/2 cup	3.0 grams
bran flakes*	3/4 cup	5.3 grams
oatmeal*, cooked	1 cup	4.0 grams
popcorn, air-popped	3 cups	3.5 grams
lentils*	1/2 cup	8 grams
lima beans*	1/2 cup	7 grams
baked beans*	1/3 cup	3.5 grams
green peas*	1/2 cup	4.4 grams
navy beans*	1/2 cup	6 grams
kidney beans*	1/2 cup	6 grams
broccoli	1/2 cup	2.6 grams
brussels sprouts*	1/2 cup	3.0 grams

Day 37

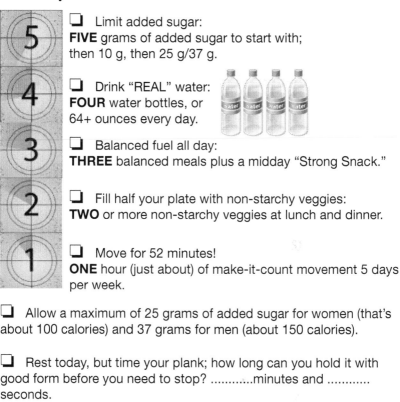

❏ Limit added sugar:
FIVE grams of added sugar to start with;
then 10 g, then 25 g/37 g.

❏ Drink "REAL" water:
FOUR water bottles, or
64+ ounces every day.

❏ Balanced fuel all day:
THREE balanced meals plus a midday "Strong Snack."

❏ Fill half your plate with non-starchy veggies:
TWO or more non-starchy veggies at lunch and dinner.

❏ Move for 52 minutes!
ONE hour (just about) of make-it-count movement 5 days
per week.

❏ Allow a maximum of 25 grams of added sugar for women (that's
about 100 calories) and 37 grams for men (about 150 calories).

❏ Rest today, but time your plank; how long can you hold it with
good form before you need to stop? ....minutes and ....
seconds.

This program has helped me greatly. Not only
do I have a new outlook on health and am
actually seeing the pounds come off, but I have
had an ever-present sense of accountability
during the Countdown.

I have a whole new outlook.

Tiphiknee, 22

Okay, time to change up your workout! Small changes count.
Unless you are doing something different every time you exercise,
something needs to change every few weeks. How? A simple
option is to change the terrain, incline, speed, or intensity. Or, try a
personal trainer or a new fitness class. Guided workouts are ideal - it
helps to have someone motivating you and checking your form (and
attendance). Even if you have a favorite sport or activity, think about

how you can vary it.

Are you logging 52 minutes, 5 days a week on Appendix D? ....
If you haven't been as consistent as you had hoped, why not move
your workout to a different time of day? Or, look into a sport or class
you've always thought of trying. The options are endless. You have
to enjoy the activity, and change it up occasionally, if you want to stay
committed to exercise with the goal of becoming "lifelong strong."

❏   I am going to change my workout by

....

....

❏   Write out your exercise plan for the week here:

SUN	
MON	
TUE	
WED	
THU	
FRI	
SAT	

Day 36

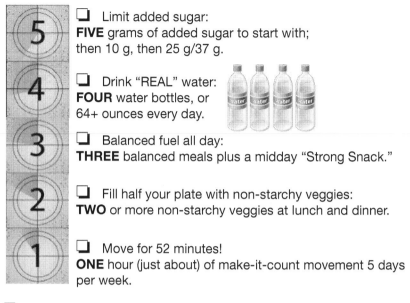

❑ Limit added sugar:
FIVE grams of added sugar to start with; then 10 g, then 25 g/37 g.

❑ Drink "REAL" water:
FOUR water bottles, or 64+ ounces every day.

❑ Balanced fuel all day:
THREE balanced meals plus a midday "Strong Snack."

❑ Fill half your plate with non-starchy veggies:
TWO or more non-starchy veggies at lunch and dinner.

❑ Move for 52 minutes!
ONE hour (just about) of make-it-count movement 5 days per week.

❑ Allow a maximum of 25 grams of added sugar for women (that's about 100 calories) and 37 grams for men (about 150 calories).

Day 36...what's $36 per week? Beyond grocery dollars, my nutrition clients tend to easily spend at least $36 on extra food and drinks for themselves each week. For example:
• $14 on 2 lunches out this week
• $6 on 2 or 3 quick coffee breaks over the week
• $12 on a dinner entrée
• $4 for a couple of sodas, Gatorades, or energy drinks during the week

It adds up quickly to $36+ per week; that's close to $2000 a year! Not to mention all those extra calories from sugary beverages and foods that most likely have more salt and fat than you would ever add at home.

Think back over the last 5 days of your week. Jot down quickly what you have spent on food for yourself (outside of your groceries):

breakfast: ………

lunches: ………

dinners: ………

drinks, coffees, vending machine beverages: ………

Estimate the total: $ ………

If you choose water over drinks that rack up, and plan well enough that you don't have to eat out as much, what could you do with that cash when it adds up over a year's time?

....

....

It will definitely provide you with some songs for your workout playlist, new athletic shoes when you need them, a consult with a registered dietitian, and a workout membership. You would have the extra dollars to buy fresh veggies and lean meats instead of being spent on padding (fat tissue) that comes from high fat, high calorie restaurant food. A healthy lifestyle doesn't have to be more expensive. But, if you find it is more, just borrow dollars from the categories noted in the bulleted examples. Both your body and your budget will thank you!

❑ Get a small envelope to keep in your car/wallet and write across it **"My food cash: $_____/week."** There are 5 weeks left from today, so each week, put in the total amount of cash you have determined is acceptable for you to spend on food and drinks for yourself (outside of your weekly grocery trip). When it runs out, it runs out...Experience is our best teacher, right?

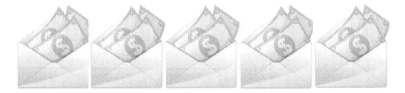

Day 35

❑ Allow a maximum of 25 grams of added sugar for women (that's about 100 calories) and 37 grams for men (about 150 calories).

Though the exact percentages have not been agreed upon by experts in the nutrition and exercise industry, most wellness professionals agree that changing your diet will make a greater impact on your weight than adding exercise. Of course, doing both is the best choice for many reasons!

5 ❑ Limit added sugar:
FIVE grams of added sugar to start with;
then 10 g, then 25 g/37 g.

4 ❑ Drink "REAL" water:
FOUR water bottles, or
64+ ounces every day.

3 ❑ Balanced fuel all day:
THREE balanced meals plus a midday "Strong Snack."

2 ❑ Fill half your plate with non-starchy veggies:
TWO or more non-starchy veggies at lunch and dinner.

1 ❑ Move for 52 minutes!
ONE hour (just about) of make-it-count movement 5 days per week.

List at least three benefits you have come to appreciate from exercise other than burning calories:

....

....

I once taught a Zumba class and went out to eat with a few of the ladies afterwards. We had just given it our all, with drenched tank tops and hair matted to our faces to prove it. It felt good to burn those 500-ish calories! I wasn't sure if they wanted me to tell them their cheese dip (not EVEN with the chips) was twice the cost of the workout they just planned their whole evening around. Tomorrow's boot camp would still just barely burn off the chips that went with the dip! There's no chance for your body to burn up those fat tissue stores if there is never a deficit of calories.

You can easily eat in 10 minutes what it takes an hour to burn off.

Calorie-dense foods quickly add up to more than you have time to work off. So even if they are healthy, they need to be limited. Some examples of calorie-dense foods include sweetened beverages, juice (limit even 100% juice to 4 ounces per day), breads at restaurants, peanut butter/nuts, cereals, alcoholic beverages, cheese, chips, fried foods, sweets, and pizza.

❑ From the list above, circle any of the calorie-dense foods or beverages that you eat.

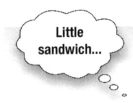

Little sandwich...

When I go to Subway, I just get the "little sandwich" (6-inch).

Mike, 59

A lot of times, people think if they choose the better-for-you option offered at a restaurant, it's automatically a good choice. It certainly may be a better choice than the alternative on the menu, but often it is much more than one would eat at home. For example, a 12-inch sub is like making three sandwiches at home (equivalent to six slices of bread plus trimmings). The bread of a 6-inch sub is equivalent to about three slices of bread. Would you eat as much bread if you were making your sandwich at home? ....

List at least five calorie-dense foods that you need to avoid or limit:

....

....

....

....

❏ If any of those foods tempt you to eat more than you would if they were not around, move them to where you can no longer access them. If your spouse or roommate insists that they stay, write their name and "FOR.................ONLY" across the opening of the package with a Sharpie in CAPS, and put them in an opaque container or bag on a high shelf, so you will not even hear them calling out to you.

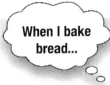

When I bake bread...

When I bake bread or goodies, I always give half of it away immediately so there is less of the tempting food for me to eat.

Kelly, 39

❏ Look back to Day 51 on page 43 and put an "X" over any entries that you are still allowing to have influence over you. Re-commit on those!

Day 34

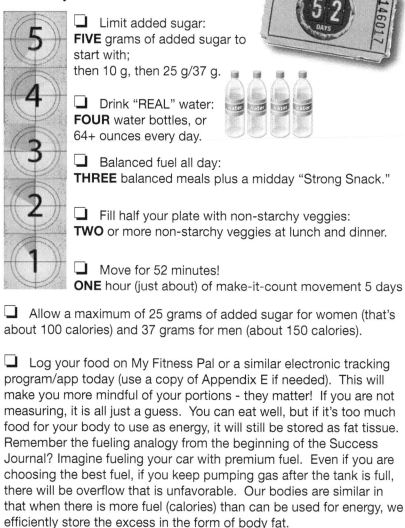

❏ Limit added sugar:
FIVE grams of added sugar to start with;
then 10 g, then 25 g/37 g.

❏ Drink "REAL" water:
FOUR water bottles, or 64+ ounces every day.

❏ Balanced fuel all day:
THREE balanced meals plus a midday "Strong Snack."

❏ Fill half your plate with non-starchy veggies:
TWO or more non-starchy veggies at lunch and dinner.

❏ Move for 52 minutes!
ONE hour (just about) of make-it-count movement 5 days

❏ Allow a maximum of 25 grams of added sugar for women (that's about 100 calories) and 37 grams for men (about 150 calories).

❏ Log your food on My Fitness Pal or a similar electronic tracking program/app today (use a copy of Appendix E if needed). This will make you more mindful of your portions - they matter! If you are not measuring, it is all just a guess. You can eat well, but if it's too much food for your body to use as energy, it will still be stored as fat tissue. Remember the fueling analogy from the beginning of the Success Journal? Imagine fueling your car with premium fuel. Even if you are choosing the best fuel, if you keep pumping gas after the tank is full, there will be overflow that is unfavorable. Our bodies are similar in that when there is more fuel (calories) than can be used for energy, we efficiently store the excess in the form of body fat.

If you are like many who sit in front of me for nutrition consults, you might say "I did so good with only a small breakfast on the early part of the day...I got busy, so I wasn't even really hungry for lunch...I came home starving and before I knew it the fridge and pantry doors were flung open... and I ate too much...I can't believe I binged on things that aren't even my favorites before I ever sat down for dinner. Then, of course, I was a little too full to finish that, so later I was hungry while watching TV, and the next thing I knew I was eating/drinking .... (fill in your late night temptation here). So, this morning I just skipped breakfast and lunch to make up for it and I'll do better tonight!"

Often that late night temptation is buttery popcorn, leftover pizza, or ice cream. Or maybe the guy from "My Favorite Pizza Place" happens to appear at your door, and you go to bed feeling defeated. If you can relate to this scenario, don't be fooled; tomorrow will look very similar if you don't break the vicious cycle of fueling poorly by day and making up for it by night.

❏ As you go along logging your food today, make sure you balance your calories so that you consume 75% of your day's total calories before 5 PM. That means that your breakfast, lunch, and "Strong Snack" need to be digested well before dinner! Don't let the hungry-monster make you crazy. Overly hungry people eat things that they often regret (and your friends and family say you are grumpy then, too).

❏ Go back to Day 46 and review the "Strong Snacks." Plan ahead to make sure those "Strong Snacks" happen daily without fail. If you are looking for something more convenient, another option that works similarly to the "Strong Snack" is just to eat half of each of the three sections off a large lunch plate, and refrigerate the other half to eat mid-afternoon. Or, consider a protein shake or a protein bar containing 150-200 calories, paired with a cup of milk or a piece of fruit.

"Strong Snack" Shakes
Monster Shake

Serves 1

Place into your blender in this order: 1/2 cup milk, 1/2 cup peach low fat Greek yogurt, 1/4 cup 100% apple juice or grape juice, 3 frozen peach wedges (or fresh), 1/2 cup ice, and a handful of baby spinach (about 1 cup of leaves), raw and washed.
Blend on high until smooth. Drink promptly.

Nutrient Breakdown (using 1% milk): Calories 196, Fat 2 g, Carb 34 g, Fiber 2 g, Protein 12 g. I suggest pairing this with a serving or two of nuts from the chart on Day 46 in order to bump up the fat and fiber to round out your "Strong Snack."

Monkey Shake

Serves 1

Place into your blender in this order: 1 cup milk, 1/2 banana, 1/2 cup ice, 1 teaspoon cocoa, 1/4 cup vanilla Greek yogurt (or 1/4 cup fat free cottage cheese) and 1 1/2 teaspoons creamy peanut butter.   Blend on high until smooth.

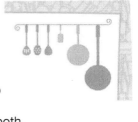

Nutrient Breakdown: Calories 259, Fat 8 g, Carb 32 g, Fiber 3 g, Protein 17 g

What would I say if I was to review your food log for today? Jot down any changes you think I would suggest. ....
....

Did eating 75% of your calories by 5:00 pm impact your evening food choices or cravings? ....

Could you continue to eat three-quarters of your calories before 5:00 pm regularly, somewhat "spoiling" your potentially voracious evening appetite with healthful foods? If so, write out a quick plan with steps to make it happen:

....
....
....

Day 33

5 ❑ Limit added sugar:
FIVE grams of added sugar to start with; then 10 g, then 25 g/37 g.

4 ❑ Drink "REAL" water:
FOUR water bottles, or 64+ ounces every day.

3 ❑ Balanced fuel all day:
THREE balanced meals plus a midday "Strong Snack."

2 ❑ Fill half your plate with non-starchy veggies:
TWO or more non-starchy veggies at lunch and dinner.

1 ❑ Move for 52 minutes!
ONE hour (just about) of make-it-count movement 5 days per week.

❏ Allow a maximum of 25 grams of added sugar for women (that's about 100 calories) and 37 grams for men (about 150 calories).

❏ REST from vigorous exercise today, but make sure you are on your feet being active at least 52 minutes of the day.

❏ Time your plank. How long can you hold it with good form before you need to stop? ....minutes and ....seconds

Remember before you started this when you looked your accountability partner in the eyes and said, "We CAN do this, you and me?" Well, is he/she still standing (running, rather) beside you? I hope so! This is essential! If not, reach out to your partner to reconnect, or recruit someone new today to complete this journey with you!

I need accountability

I am going to do the Countdown with my Zumba class even though I recently met my weight goal. I have learned I must have ongoing accountability to keep it off.

Nicole, 44

❏ It is time to call or visit your accountability partner, or get together for a walk (a nice stroll is okay on a "rest day" for an active person like you). No texts or emails on this one, please. Believe it or not, it will be more motivating for you to hear his/her actual voice encouraging you!

❏ Please cover the following in your conversation:
1) Report three successes:

....

....

2) Discuss challenges and ask for feedback.
Challenges to discuss: ....

....

Feedback from my partner: ....

....

3) Share a commitment you will make between now and the next check-in.

....

....

4) Decide on a consequence and a reward for each other related to those commitments. For example: "Let's go play golf, or go get a pedicure on Saturday if we are able to.................................all week." Or "If I don't walk/run 3 miles with you 3 times this week, I will wash your car by hand."

Reward:...

Consequence:...

Day 32

❑ Limit added sugar:
FIVE grams of added sugar to start with; then 10 g, then 25 g/37 g.

❑ Drink "REAL" water:
FOUR water bottles, or 64+ ounces every day.

❑ Balanced fuel all day:
THREE balanced meals plus a midday "Strong Snack."

❑ Fill half your plate with non-starchy veggies:
TWO or more non-starchy veggies at lunch and dinner.

❑ Move for 52 minutes!
ONE hour (just about) of make-it-count movement 5 days per week.

❑ Allow a maximum of 25 grams of added sugar for women (that's about 100 calories) and 37 grams for men (about 150 calories).

About a third of the calories American adults and children consume are from restaurants and other food-service establishments outside the home. Over the same decades that obesity prevalence has tripled, the frequency of eating out has increased dramatically.

Multiple studies have shown that eating out more frequently is associated with higher body fatness, obesity, and higher body mass index. Women who eat out more than 5 meals a week consume nearly 300 more calories per day than women who eat out less often. That adds up to about 10 pounds of extra padding every 4 months.

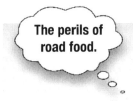

The perils of road food.

I just started a new job with a lot of travel involved and I have gained 10 pounds in just three months!

Anonymous, 24

Even if consumers start making better food choices when eating out, they still tend to take in more fat and calories, and eat larger portions then they would otherwise. I advise my clients to set a limit on the number of meals that they eat out (ideally no more than 2-3 meals/week).

Considering the research and your current dining out habits, how many meals should you set as your dining out limit per week?
My goal for maximum number of meals I eat out per week:
Breakfasts: .... Lunches: .... Dinners:.................
Keep using the envelopes as suggested on Day 36, and the limit to available funds for eating out will help keep you committed.

PLACES I GO OUT TO EAT	WHAT I EAT WHEN I'M THERE	✔	WHAT I'M GOING TO EAT INSTEAD

"Check" the column after looking up the nutrition information.

Dangerous restaurants for my health: (circle)
buffet   fast food   gourmet food   sandwich shop   bar & grill
Italian   Asian   Mexican   French

96

Day 31

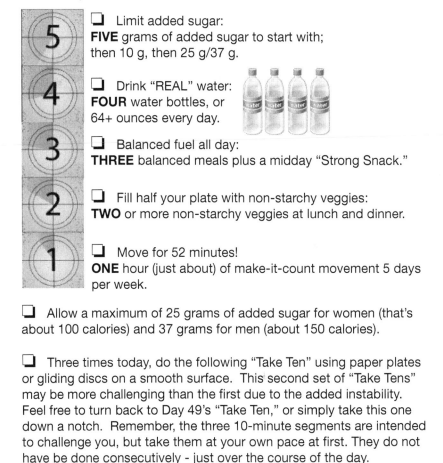

❏ Limit added sugar:
FIVE grams of added sugar to start with; then 10 g, then 25 g/37 g.

❏ Drink "REAL" water:
FOUR water bottles, or 64+ ounces every day.

❏ Balanced fuel all day:
THREE balanced meals plus a midday "Strong Snack."

❏ Fill half your plate with non-starchy veggies:
TWO or more non-starchy veggies at lunch and dinner.

❏ Move for 52 minutes!
ONE hour (just about) of make-it-count movement 5 days per week.

❏ Allow a maximum of 25 grams of added sugar for women (that's about 100 calories) and 37 grams for men (about 150 calories).

❏ Three times today, do the following "Take Ten" using paper plates or gliding discs on a smooth surface. This second set of "Take Tens" may be more challenging than the first due to the added instability. Feel free to turn back to Day 49's "Take Ten," or simply take this one down a notch. Remember, the three 10-minute segments are intended to challenge you, but take them at your own pace at first. They do not have be done consecutively - just over the course of the day.

Take Ten

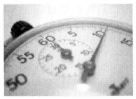

Minute 1: hold a plank on your hands instead of forearms, and with your toes on the plates, draw each knee in alternately to opposite elbow while keeping hips down and naval pressed to spine, hovering over the floor

curtsey lunge

Minute 2: curtsey lunges with ball of each foot sliding the plate back, alternating right and left with fairly quick tempo (see photo)

Minute 3: 30 seconds of push-ups, 30 seconds of triceps dips

Minute 4: stand on the plates on your toes, feet together, and do a quick hip twist side to side, pushing one arm out at a time in front of you as your upper body twists opposite of your lower body

Minute 5: with the ball of each foot on a plate, do lateral shuffles (quick shuffle steps sideways across the room and back)

Minute 6: scissor shuffle - toes pointing forward, plates under feet in tandem foot position, switching feet in a scissoring motion; arms like you're running

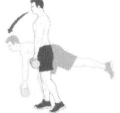

single-leg deadlift

Minute 7: stand as wide as you can on the plates, toes out and hips low: 1) bring feet together with a quick hop, standing taller as you draw feet in; 2) slide out with a little scoot and repeat (as you get more comfortable with this, you can do it more briskly)

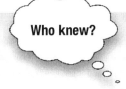

mountain climber

Minute 8: single-leg dead lift (weighted if desired), 10 R, 10 L and repeat (see above)

Minute 9: "mountain climbers" with balls of feet on discs/plates (see photo, left)

Minute 10: basic crunches (exhale on lift)

Take a quick break between each minute if needed. These are meant to be tough for every fitness level, so don't get discouraged if you are new, or deconditioned.

Be sure to take a few minutes to cool-down and stretch afterwards. Use the following link if you need a guide for stretching: http://www.mayoclinic.com/health/stretching/SM00043&slide=2

❏   Email or text your partner: "I did Day 31's 'Take Ten' three times today, and it was ....!"

Who knew?   Who knew a seemingly harmless paper plate could create such a challenging workout!

Jimmieann, 36

Day 30

5 ❏ Limit added sugar:
FIVE grams of added sugar to start with; then 10 g, then 25 g/37 g.

4 ❏ Drink "REAL" water:
FOUR water bottles, or 64+ ounces every day.

3 ❏ Balanced fuel all day:
THREE balanced meals plus a midday "Strong Snack."

2 ❏ Fill half your plate with non-starchy veggies:
TWO or more non-starchy veggies at lunch and dinner.

1 ❏ Move for 52 minutes!
ONE hour (just about) of make-it-count movement 5 days per week.

❏ Allow a maximum of 25 grams of added sugar for women (that's about 100 calories) and 37 grams for men (about 150 calories).

❏ REST from vigorous exercise today, but make sure you are on your feet being active at least 52 minutes of the day.

❏ Time your plank. How long can you hold it with good form before you need to stop? ....minutes and ....seconds

After having a couple of days to think about how many calories go in when you eat out, let's talk about planning! Do you ever eat out just because you feel like you have to for the sake of time or energy? Have you ever heard, "Failure to plan is a plan to fail?" It is so true! The type of food you need to eat to reach Your Best Body doesn't just end up on your table, or even in your refrigerator...and you don't typically just happen by the gym in workout clothes, do you?

It takes as much energy to wish as it does to plan.
— Eleanor Roosevelt

Have you made a menu for this week? Do you know which days you are exercising? Where, and with whom? When are you eating out next, and what you will eat? If you find meal planning daunting and you need a little help, check out bestbodyin52.com for recipes and "Indestructible" for meal plans.

❏ Using the following Meal Planning worksheet, write out a menu plan of dinners for the week, including any dining out plans. Don't let meals sneak up on you! Feel free to do the same for breakfast and lunch if you like. Appendix G has an extra copy of this chart for your convenience, and it is also available on my website.

❏ Take a picture of the completed table below and email or text it to

MEAL PLANNING	PICTURE IT!	GROCERY NEEDS	PREPARATION TIPS
Monday's Dinner			
Tuesday's Dinner			
Wednesday's Dinner			
Thursday's Dinner			
Friday's Dinner			
Saturday's Dinner			
Sunday's Dinner			

your partner, and also to your wellness coordinator/coach if applicable.

Pita Pizza

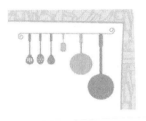

Serves 4

Perfect for a fun lunch or a super-quick dinner, and always a hit with kids!

4 whole wheat pita rounds
1 cup mozzarella cheese
1/4 cup pizza sauce
1 1/2 cups fresh spinach, chopped
2 teaspoons fresh basil leaves, chopped
1/4 cup red onions, chopped
1 cup fresh tomatoes, chopped
1 cup red bell peppers, chopped
1 small can of sliced olives (2.25 ounces)
1 teaspoon dried oregano (about 1/4 teaspoon per pizza)
24 turkey pepperoni rounds (about 6 rounds per pizza)

1. Preheat oven to 400 degrees. Set four whole wheat round pitas on a cookie sheet.
2. Spoon 1 tablespoon of your favorite pizza/pasta sauce on each.
3. Add chopped spinach and basil.
4. Reserving 2 tablespoons to add at the end, spoon 2 tablespoons of mozzarella cheese on each pita round. Add any of the veggies above as desired.
5. Sprinkle the reserved 2 tablespoons of cheese over each pita round and add oregano.
6. Cut turkey pepperoni rounds in quarters and place over the pizza.
7. Bake at 400 degrees for 7-10 minutes, or until cheese is bubbly and edges are browning.

Nutrient Breakdown: Calories 281, Fat 10 g, (4 g Sat. Fat), Sodium 752 mg, Carbohydrate 35 g, Fiber 6 g, Protein 16 g

Day 29

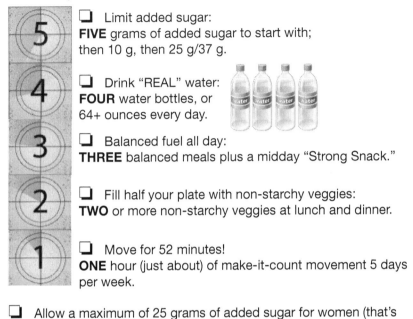

❏ Limit added sugar:
FIVE grams of added sugar to start with; then 10 g, then 25 g/37 g.

❏ Drink "REAL" water:
FOUR water bottles, or 64+ ounces every day.

❏ Balanced fuel all day:
THREE balanced meals plus a midday "Strong Snack."

❏ Fill half your plate with non-starchy veggies:
TWO or more non-starchy veggies at lunch and dinner.

❏ Move for 52 minutes!
ONE hour (just about) of make-it-count movement 5 days per week.

❏ Allow a maximum of 25 grams of added sugar for women (that's about 100 calories) and 37 grams for men (about 150 calories).

"29 and holding?" Did you know that your age has less impact on your fitness level than your commitment level? Plenty of teenagers huff and puff in my fitness classes more than the 60 year old regulars in the back row who can hold a plank for 2 plus minutes with no problem.

We all know that to a certain degree, aging comes with limitations, but don't let your gray hairs hold you back! I am pushing 40 and am leaner than when I was in my 20s...I even ran my fastest 5k recently. I have no boastful intentions, I am just saying that staying this course WORKS! I live this out every 52 days and you can too!

Recently, a girl at the gym said to me, "Good to see you. You look great." (That's what girls say in the South when they haven't seen you in awhile, regardless of how you look. I am not one to get fixed up to go to the gym). Then she said, looking me up and down in my sweat-soaked gym clothes, "Well, you look the same. You always look the same - except your hair is longer."

As you reach Your Best Body, plan not to adjust your belt notches ever again. Seriously - it is possible! Imagine what the New Year would be like without a resolution in this department. A 3-5 pound fluctuation is reasonable from now on. Let it be the new, lifelong shape of you.

Mark an "X" below to show where you think you stand on this continuum:

| I doubt I can maintain this | Maybe a 10-pound range | I'll stay within a 3 to 5 pound range |

❑ Fill in the blank: When this 52 day Countdown concludes, I'm going to

....

....

I hope it says, "Start the 52 days anew with another accountability partner to encourage along the way!" Or, "Join INDESTRUCTIBLE and do another 52 days with even more tools for success!"

No matter how big your goal is, it is not impossible! Take one day, one week, and one month at a time and you will see results. Never give up and you will reach your goal!

Never give up!

Becky, 34

(Becky has lost 87 pounds and has just a few more pounds to go before reaching her goal weight!)

❑ Write out Your Best Body SMART goal - to be completed in the next 29 days. To follow the SMART acronym, your goal needs to be "Specific, Measurable, Attainable, Realistic and Time-Bound." Note: if you are setting goals related to weight or body fat percentage, you need to give yourself a 3-5 pound range, or a 1-3 percent range, not an exact number. Otherwise you will simply set yourself up for frustration, as it is normal for your body to fluctuate. When the numbers change slightly, keep in mind it is not always fat tissue increasing and decreasing over the hours of the day.

What is your short term SMART goal for the remainder of the Countdown?

....

....

Write your lifelong Best Body-related SMART goal here:

....

....

....

Are both of the goals above:
- O   Specific?
- O   Measurable?
- O   Attainable?
- O   Realistic?
- O   Time-Bound?

❏   Please take a picture of your goals and email or text it to your partner.

Day 28

5 ❏   Limit added sugar:
FIVE grams of added sugar to start with; then 10 g, then 25 g/37 g.

4 ❏   Drink "REAL" water:
FOUR water bottles, or 64+ ounces every day.

3 ❏   Balanced fuel all day:
THREE balanced meals plus a midday "Strong Snack."

2 ❏   Fill half your plate with non-starchy veggies:
TWO or more non-starchy veggies at lunch and dinner.

1 ❏   Move for 52 minutes!
ONE hour (just about) of make-it-count movement 5 days per week.

❏   Allow a maximum of 25 grams of added sugar for women (that's about 100 calories) and 37 grams for men (about 150 calories).

I keep losing weight every week and I really don't even feel deprived or hungry. I have tried every diet, and the nagging hunger is usually what makes me quit. Eating healthy food rather than just calorie counting, and making sure I have a "Strong Snack" every day really makes a difference.

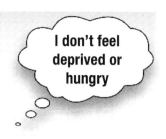

Mary, 50

Constantly hungry? I don't let any of my clients go around starving. If you are feeling hungry too often then here are some quick helps:

❑ Does your breakfast meet the "Best Body breakfast" guidelines I suggested on Day 45?

❑ Are you eating something with protein, fat, and fiber every 3-5 hours?

❑ Are you eating 3 meals and a "Strong Snack" every afternoon? Remember some people with long, active days often need two "Strong Snacks" over the course of the day.

❑ Could you be eating too fast? Take smaller bites and set your fork down between bites to take a sip of water.

❑ Are you drinking at least 64 ounces of water daily (drinking with meals as well as in between meals)?

❑ Could you be exercising excessively?

❑ Are you getting in 25-35 grams of fiber daily?

❑ Are you sleeping at least 7 hours per night?

❑ Could it be "mouth hunger" rather than true hunger? (I am instantly "hungry" if fresh baked goodies are around. You too?)

❑ Could your weight goal or your caloric intake be too low, causing you to eat less than your body truly needs?

If you are still sincerely hungry after exploring the above guidelines:
1) Discontinue any foods/gum/drinks with artificial sweeteners.
2) Increase the weight, and hence the filling-power, of your meals by adding a broth-based vegetable soup (watch the sodium).
3) Add an extra serving of fiber-rich non-starchy veggies to lunch and/or dinner if you are not satisfied.
4) If you are still hungry and it is nighttime, perhaps it is time for bed. If you are awake too long, you will naturally be hungry for another meal's worth of calories.
5) Set up a personalized consultation with a registered dietitian.

❏ Complete the following assessment at each meal and snack today to become more aware of your hunger at different times of the day, and to assess how satisfied you are after meals.

Hunger Log

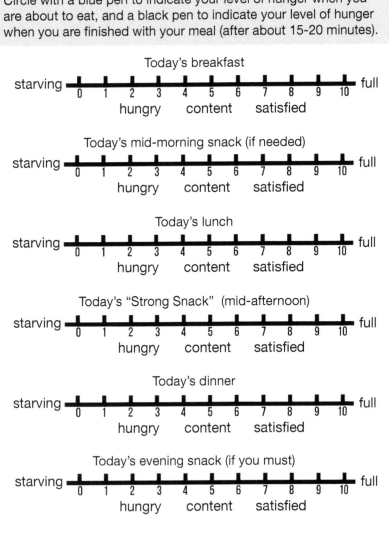

Circle with a blue pen to indicate your level of hunger when you are about to eat, and a black pen to indicate your level of hunger when you are finished with your meal (after about 15-20 minutes).

Today's breakfast

starving — 0 1 2 3 4 5 6 7 8 9 10 — full

hungry   content   satisfied

Today's mid-morning snack (if needed)

starving — 0 1 2 3 4 5 6 7 8 9 10 — full

hungry   content   satisfied

Today's lunch

starving — 0 1 2 3 4 5 6 7 8 9 10 — full

hungry   content   satisfied

Today's "Strong Snack" (mid-afternoon)

starving — 0 1 2 3 4 5 6 7 8 9 10 — full

hungry   content   satisfied

Today's dinner

starving — 0 1 2 3 4 5 6 7 8 9 10 — full

hungry   content   satisfied

Today's evening snack (if you must)

starving — 0 1 2 3 4 5 6 7 8 9 10 — full

hungry   content   satisfied

At most of your meals, you'll want to eat until you reach somewhere between "content" and "satisfied." If weight loss is your goal, at your last meal of the day, stop eating when you are "content."

Have you been logging your weight for the week on Appendix C's graph? .... Your thoughts on your progress in this area?..................
....

Day 27

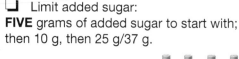

❏ Limit added sugar:
FIVE grams of added sugar to start with;
then 10 g, then 25 g/37 g.

❏ Drink "REAL" water:
FOUR water bottles, or
64+ ounces every day.

❏ Balanced fuel all day:
THREE balanced meals plus a midday "Strong Snack."

❏ Fill half your plate with non-starchy veggies:
TWO or more non-starchy veggies at lunch and dinner.

❏ Move for 52 minutes!
ONE hour (just about) of make-it-count movement 5 days per week.

❏ Allow a maximum of 25 grams of added sugar for women (that's about 100 calories) and 37 grams for men (about 150 calories).

Someone I knew in college would have what he called a "Fatterday" every weekend. Can you guess what that means? On Saturdays he would have a "cheat" day and eat absolutely whatever he wanted. Some people do that without realizing it, thinking "When I am at home I am careful, but when I'm out I just eat whatever I feel like having." If you consider any day a "cheat day" or if you eat away from home more than once a week with that perspective, it could be enough to hold you back from reaching Your Best Body.

Do you ever have a "Fatterday" on Saturdays or any other day of the week? ....If you tend to overdo it on the weekends or otherwise, your daily exercise could just be burning off your "Fatterday." Many people I have worked with invest in their gym membership and workout gear, and make the hard work of exercising happen consistently JUST to work off their weekend splurges.

"FATTERDAY"	ON TOP OF A REGULAR LUNCH & DINNER, IS SPLURGING WORTH THE COST?
Morning	4 medium pancakes with syrup **(900 calories)**
Afternoon Starbucks splurge	Venti White Chocolate Mocha (600 calories) and a banana nut loaf (490 calories) = **1090 (WHOA!)**
Date night!	You make wise choices at dinner, but for a splurge, split the "Bloomin' Onion" appetizer with your date (you get 1,065 of the 2,130 calories added to dinner) and share a medium popcorn at the movies (1,200 calories...600 are yours) = **1,665 (YIKES!)**
Total cost of one "Fatterday's" splurges	900 1090 + 1665 **3655** = NINE 52-minute workouts (is it worth it?)

Which day of the week do you tend to overeat, or "cheat?" Or, instead is it a certain time of the day?

....

Which foods are typically involved if and when you splurge?

....
....

What is your plan to keep treats or splurges from sabotaging your efforts?

....
....
....

❑   Log your food on My Fitness Pal or a similar tracking program/app today (use a copy of Appendix E if you are unable to enter it directly into an electronic tracking program or app, but be sure to transfer it as soon as you can). Would you benefit from daily food tracking for the remainder of the Countdown?.............. Will you? ....

❑ Be sure to measure each food (just for today) so you know your food log is providing you with an accurate analysis.

❑ Mark your calendar or set a reminder in your phone for the first week of every month for the next 6 months, reminding you to record food and exercise for the week. Plan to share your log with your accountability partner each month to keep yourself in check.

❑ Check in with your partner today to see if he/she marked the calendar as suggested above.

Day 26

❑ Limit added sugar:
FIVE grams of added sugar to start with; then 10 g, then 25 g/37 g.

❑ Drink "REAL" water:
FOUR water bottles, or 64+ ounces every day.

❑ Balanced fuel all day:
THREE balanced meals plus a midday "Strong Snack."

❑ Fill half your plate with non-starchy veggies:
TWO or more non-starchy veggies at lunch and dinner.

❑ Move for 52 minutes!
ONE hour (just about) of make-it-count movement 5 days per week.

❑ Allow a maximum of 25 grams of added sugar for women (that's about 100 calories) and 37 grams for men (about 150 calories).

❑ Rest from vigorous activity today, but time your plank. How long can you hold it with good form before you need to stop?
.... minutes and .... seconds

You are half-way there! Congratulations! Have you thought about how you will reward yourself when you reach your goal(s)? No, not with chocolate or a night out at your favorite restaurant or bar! Incentives help motivate, but they must not be food related.

Are you in the habit of using food or drinks as a reward or prize for yourself or others?............. If so, could this be dangerous for you?
....

Suggestions for rewards:
  • A new book or magazine and a hot bubble bath if you faithfully exercise for 52 minutes for 5 days of the week (in a 7 day period).
  • A pedicure for 10 toes if you lose 10% of your body weight.
  • Put a dollar in a jar each time you choose a healthy choice over a tempting poor choice and let it build up so you can get something fun that will promote your health, like a bicycle, or hand weights.
  • New workout clothes or shoes once you have gotten rid of all the junk food in your house and stayed away from it for two weeks.
  • Housekeeping! Hire someone to "pick up" for you once you have gone a week without "picking up" any processed food!
  • Put a golf ball in a large jar for each day you log your food and go for a round of golf with your accountability partner once it's full!

Over the next two weeks, once I am able to consistently
....,
I will reward myself with
....

When I reach my Best Body goal, I will reward myself by:
....
....

Are you recording your exercise weekly on Appendix D? ....
If not, start today or tomorrow!

110

Day 25

5 ❑ Limit added sugar:
FIVE grams of added sugar to start with;
then 10 g, then 25 g/37 g.

4 ❑ Drink "REAL" water:
FOUR water bottles, or
64+ ounces every day.

3 ❑ Balanced fuel all day:
THREE balanced meals plus a midday "Strong Snack."

2 ❑ Fill half your plate with non-starchy veggies:
TWO or more non-starchy veggies at lunch and dinner.

1 ❑ Move for 52 minutes!
ONE hour (just about) of make-it-count movement 5 days
per week.

❑ Allow a maximum of 25 grams of added sugar for women (that's
about 100 calories) and 37 grams for men (about 150 calories).

It's time to push yourself. Must. Read. On. Typically, new exercisers
can see and feel strength and endurance gains around the 4-6
week mark. You have been working at this for about 4 weeks.
Congratulations! So, it's time to take it up a notch! For example,
if you are lifting weights, it's time to go heavier. If you are jogging,
walking, or biking, it's time to go faster or add some hills. Your body
will adapt to the load you are putting on it and if it is not challenged,
you will hit a plateau.

If you have been consistent with your exercise, you should be starting
to feel a difference in stamina and strength. Do you? ....

If you have not been consistent, brainstorm below what it will take for
you to get into a routine that ensures regular exercise.

....

....

....

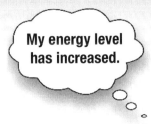

My energy level has increased.

I now swim and workout at the gym several days each week, and put movement into every part of my day. My energy level and strength have increased dramatically. My weight has gone from 226 pounds to under 200 and at age 69, I am happy to say that I now feel many years younger!

Allan, 69

❏ Today, beat all of last week's markers...even if it's just by a little. Check which of the following you can or will do starting today:

○ I can exceed my biking, walking, and/or jogging speed.
○ I can do one more pushup in the time allotted.
○ I will dance with more vigor.
○ I can leap a little higher or jump rope a little faster.
○ I can hold my plank a little longer.
○ I will add weight to exercises like walking lunges.
○ I will add a riser to my step in my aerobics class.
○ I will lift heavier weights.
○ I will walk, jog, or bike in an area with more hills or use a steeper incline.

With your partner, brainstorm which changes you both will make, together even. Use some from the list above, or come up with your own:

....

....

Be the best you can be and resist the staleness that comes when you don't challenge yourself. What did you do today to beat a previous marker?

....

....

Day 24

5 ❑ Limit added sugar:
FIVE grams of added sugar to start with; then 10 g, then 25 g/37 g.

4 ❑ Drink "REAL" water:
FOUR water bottles, or 64+ ounces every day.

3 ❑ Balanced fuel all day:
THREE balanced meals plus a midday "Strong Snack."

2 ❑ Fill half your plate with non-starchy veggies:
TWO or more non-starchy veggies at lunch and dinner.

1 ❑ Move for 52 minutes!
ONE hour (just about) of make-it-count movement 5 days per week.

❑ Allow a maximum of 25 grams of added sugar for women (that's about 100 calories) and 37 grams for men (about 150 calories).

Hmm...Day 24...4x6 is 24...Sounds like a photo op to me!
❑ Have your accountability partner take a photo of you in those same fitted workout clothes from the first photo, and have one taken together. Compare them to your start-up photos by posting them at the beginning of your Success Journal. Seeing the difference is motivating!

How do you feel about your progress so far?

....

....

FAQ

Q: I'm getting leaner, but should I feel this tired?

A: Readers following the daily guidelines of the Countdown, and taking on new healthy habits from what they've learned as they go, typically do not suffer from fatigue or a lack of energy during the program. If you are feeling low in energy, however, consider the following. Check any that may alert you to what you need to change.

113

O Are you drinking at least 64 ounces of water daily?

O Are you getting at **least** 1200-1400 calories, or more if you are active and, per my fueling analogy, "drive a larger car" or always moving with your "pedal to the metal."

O Could you be over-doing your exercise or skipping your rest days? Everyone needs at least 1 rest day per week.

O Are you avoiding any of the major food groups? (If you are "picky," be sure to take a multivitamin as a back-up and refer to Day 21's recommendations).

O Are you getting good quality sleep at night for at least 7 hours?

O Are you anemic or low in iron? (Ask your healthcare provider for a blood test to determine if you need extra supplementation).

Day 23

❏ Limit added sugar:
FIVE grams of added sugar to start with; then 10 g, then 25 g/37 g.

❏ Drink "REAL" water:
FOUR water bottles, or 64+ ounces every day.

❏ Balanced fuel all day:
THREE balanced meals plus a midday "Strong Snack."

❏ Fill half your plate with non-starchy veggies:
TWO or more non-starchy veggies at lunch and dinner.

❏ Move for 52 minutes!
ONE hour (just about) of make-it-count movement 5 days per week.

❏ Allow a maximum of 25 grams of added sugar for women (that's about 100 calories) and 37 grams for men (about 150 calories).

❏ Rest today, but time your plank; how long can you hold it with good form before you need to stop? ....minutes and ....seconds.

So, now that you are over the halfway hump, to which lifestyle change(s) do you assign the most credit for your Best-Body progress?

....

....

....

What could still be holding you back? (The most common answers I hear from my clients are: drinking alcohol, eating out too much, allowing tempting foods in my house, failing to plan ahead, and letting other things take priority over exercise).

....

....

....

To overcome any setback(s), list two affirming statements below about your capability to do well over the rest of the Countdown. Write out the truth of what you know you have the potential to do, clearly dispelling any discouraging lies you may be tempted to believe.

....

....

....

....

If you need renewed focus, zone in on the strategies below. These have made the biggest impact in the lives of those that I work with weekly.

Check the ones below that you feel great about, and highlight three to which you need to give more attention.

○ Limit added sugar to a maximum of 25 grams/day for women (100 calories), or 37 for men (150 calories), ideally not from beverages.

○ Water! Water! Water! (Are you great at this yet?)

○ Eat 3 balanced meals and a "Strong Snack" in the afternoon, and an additional "Strong Snack" if necessary.

○ Make sure that half your plate is non-starchy veggies at lunch and supper.

○ Log food daily into an online tracking program like My Fitness Pal right after each meal, or even just before. (Those who keep track of their daily intake have great success).

○ Move for 52 minutes, and make sure at least half the time has you perspiring!

❏ Take a moment to look over previous days in your Success Journal to recall what I mean by "strong" and "clean." (See Day 46 and Day 38, respectively). Describe the following in your own words:

"Strong" (as in "strong snack")

....

....

"Clean" (as in "clean eating")

....

....

❏ Look back to find your first plank time from the start-up assessment (....................) and compare it to today's time (....................). Thoughts?

....

Have you stayed committed to doing the plank exercise twice a week as suggested in the Countdown? If so, what benefits have you gained?

....

....

If not, how can you intentionally schedule this into your routine at least twice a week?

....

....

Day 22

5 ❑ Limit added sugar:
FIVE grams of added sugar to start with;
then 10 g, then 25 g/37 g.

4 ❑ Drink "REAL" water:
FOUR water bottles, or
64+ ounces every day.

3 ❑ Balanced fuel all day:
THREE balanced meals plus a midday "Strong Snack."

2 ❑ Fill half your plate with non-starchy veggies:
TWO or more non-starchy veggies at lunch and dinner.

1 ❑ Move for 52 minutes!
ONE hour (just about) of make-it-count movement 5 days
per week.

❑ Allow a maximum of 25 grams of added sugar for women (that's about 100 calories) and 37 grams for men (about 150 calories).

Did you know that an extra 100 calories per day add up to 10 pounds of fat tissue by the end of the year? It doesn't take too many extra sips or bites, especially if the food is fried, creamy, or sweet.

Many of us grew up finishing every bite served on our plates, or finishing the last serving in the dish just because it's there, without regarding our level of hunger or fullness. Do you feel guilty if you leave a few bites on the plate? Unfortunately, eating those extra bites does not help those in need of food, instead it harms your body.

What can you do to change this lose-lose situation to a win-win?

....

....

Explore any reasons (other than hunger) why you may find yourself eating unnecessarily, and possibly even overeating:

117

"Even if I am not hungry, I tend to eat when I am ...." (check)

○ bored
○ stressed
○ celebrating/happy
○ sad
○ at family gatherings
○ going to events where food is offered (ex: movies after dinner)
○ near accessible food
○ staying up too late/tired/sleep deprived
○ watching TV
○ drinking alcohol
○ other:...............................

A meta-analysis of 23 studies measured if people tended to eat more when engaged in the last three listed above. Researchers found that of the three, alcohol (typically 1 to 2 1/2 servings) most impacts the number of servings you eat, followed by sleep deprivation (less than 5 1/2 hours vs. 8 or more hours), and then watching enticing food images on the screen (for about 25 to 45 minutes, per this research). All three may also impact your inhibitions, thus leading to choices you would not have otherwise made.

Review what you checked off above and think through how you can set yourself up for success now that you've identified some eating triggers other than hunger. For example, thank your family for all the goodies they bring over for dinner, but let them know that you need them to take their leftovers home.

Plan to be especially mindful of your intake today:
❏ Put a reminder in your phone/watch that will go off at mealtimes reminding you to eat slowly and mindfully.
❏ Anticipate the flavors of each food you eat and chew intentionally, putting your fork down in between bites.
❏ Eat slowly enough to give your body the chance to signal you when you are satisfied.
❏ Refrigerate or freeze extras rather than "cleaning" your plate. If you tend to have quite a bit of waste, consider buying and making less food and donating the dollars you save in doing so to an agency serving the needy.

Whatever you do, do not let your mouth be where you "dispose" of extra food! You can be sure your body will not waste food - those bites will be saved securely in the form of fat cells on your ....
(note the most likely location on your body for those extra calories to accumulate into pounds).

Whatever you do, do not let your mouth be where you "dispose" of extra food!

Day 21

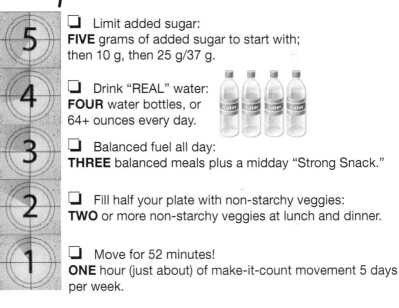

5 ❑ Limit added sugar:
FIVE grams of added sugar to start with;
then 10 g, then 25 g/37 g.

4 ❑ Drink "REAL" water:
FOUR water bottles, or
64+ ounces every day.

3 ❑ Balanced fuel all day:
THREE balanced meals plus a midday "Strong Snack."

2 ❑ Fill half your plate with non-starchy veggies:
TWO or more non-starchy veggies at lunch and dinner.

1 ❑ Move for 52 minutes!
ONE hour (just about) of make-it-count movement 5 days per week.

❑ Allow a maximum of 25 grams of added sugar for women (that's about 100 calories) and 37 grams for men (about 150 calories).

So you are eating healthily and exercising regularly...is that enough? Does your diet need supplementation? If you are eating a low calorie diet (under 1600 calories/day), or if you typically are not getting a variety of foods from all the food groups, then it is a good idea to use a multivitamin/multimineral supplement as a back-up. It's generally safer to do this than to take several individual vitamins. Often times, too much of a good thing is not a "good thing" nutritionally. See Appendix H for recommendations.

There are a few supplements worth taking in addition to your multi:

❑ Count up your **calcium**. Think through what you ate yesterday and the day before. How many servings did you take in from milk, yogurt, cheese or a calcium-fortified dairy-alternative? (Refer to Day 45 for the servings sizes of calcium-rich foods.) ....

On average, if you do not take in 3-4 servings per day of calcium-rich foods or beverages, each containing 300-400 mg of calcium, then you may need a supplement. The Recommended Daily Allowance (RDA) for 19-50 year old adults is 1000 mg and bumps up to 1200 mg for women over 51 years of age and men over 71. There is typically not enough calcium in a multivitamin to make up for a lack of dairy consumption at most meals. Due to research on male subjects regarding increased risk for both heart disease and prostate cancer, I recommend no more than 400 mg of supplemented calcium for men daily. Men typically meet their calcium needs through their daily intake more readily than women, so simply adding a multivitamin for back-up is sufficient. For women, at each meal that does not contain one of the calcium-rich foods noted previously, I recommend a supplement containing 300-500 mg of calcium (ideally just 1 or 2 times daily).

If you are drinking calcium fortified beverages in addition to calcium-rich foods, it is possible to get too much, especially for men. Conversely, if you think you are meeting your calcium needs from greens, you are most likely not getting enough, as it takes 3 cups of broccoli, for example, to get the calcium in one cup of milk.

Even where there is plenty of sunshine, many people are testing low for **Vitamin D.** The Institute of Medicine recommendation has been increased to 600 IU a day for adults up to age 70 and 800 IU for people over 70.

❑ Make sure to eat a variety of foods so you can get some of your Vitamin D from eggs; salmon and other fatty fish; and fortified foods like milk, breakfast cereals, some brands of yogurt and orange juice. If you eat a variety of these foods daily, you may be able to meet your needs along with the support of a basic daily multivitamin, which typically contains about 400 IU of vitamin D. However, many people need the supplementation, so if you are in doubt talk to your doctor about taking the additional vitamin D supplement.

Omega-3s: Taking in omega-3 fatty acids may have a variety of benefits, from decreasing inflammation to improving triglycerides in the blood. In short, it's best to get your omega-3s from at least two palm-sized portions per week of fatty fish like salmon, trout, herring, flounder, mackerel or albacore tuna. If you are intentional, you may also get some omega-3s from canola oil, walnuts, soybeans, and flaxseeds, as well as fortified foods available in grocery stores as of late. Taking a supplement of 1000-1200 mg EPA+DHA is a great back-up. Greater doses may be recommended based on your medical history, but intake of greater than 3 grams may cause excessive bleeding in some people, so be sure to talk to your healthcare provider.

❏ Check here if you will have or have had at least one of the omega-3 sources above today. Keeping this up may make a difference in many facets of your long term health! If you do not regularly eat omega-rich foods, how can you improve your intake?

....

....

The following recipes go together beautifully. Serve the Broiled Salmon over the Super-Food Salad with The Perfect Dressing. Add a side of Pita Chips from the recipe on Day 15, if desired.

Broiled Salmon

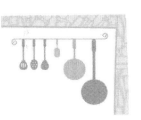

Serves 4-6

16-20 ounces of salmon (choose wild salmon over farmed)
1/4 cup lemon juice
2 teaspoons olive oil
1 tablespoon Mrs. Dash Garlic and Herb variety
1/4 teaspoon Cavender's Greek seasoning
dill, as desired

1. Mix lemon juice, oil, and seasonings together.
2. Drizzle that mix over a shallow foil-covered baking dish.
3. Dip salmon into the liquid and seasonings on both sides until covered.

4. Sprinkle dill over the top of each salmon filet as desired.
Broil for 4-7 minutes on each side, depending on the thickness of the fish. When turning the salmon, remove skin easily by sliding a spatula under the skin and add more dill when fish is flipped.

Nutrient Breakdown: Calories: 189, Fat 7 g, (1 g Sat. Fat), Sodium 459 mg, Carbohydrate 2 g, Fiber 0 g, Protein 28 g

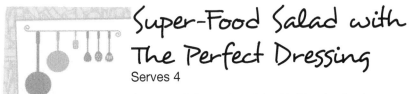

Super-Food Salad with The Perfect Dressing
Serves 4

4 cups rainbow slaw (aka California slaw), chopped slightly
1 pint cherry or grape tomatoes, halved
6 cups baby spinach leaves, washed

The Perfect Dressing

1 large garlic clove
Fresh cracked pepper to taste
1/8 teaspoon salt
2 tablespoons lemon juice
1 tablespoon olive oil
1-2 fresh basil leaves, finely chopped, if desired

1. In a large bowl, mix the first 3 salad ingredients.
2. Process garlic into a paste using a mortar and pestle, or the back of a spoon after mincing the garlic.
3. Add salt and pepper to garlic paste and further process it until combined well.
4. Mix the paste into a cup with the lemon juice and olive oil.
5. Add fresh basil if desired and mix well.
6. Toss into the bowl with the veggies, stirring well until covered.
Caution: a very small amount of this dressing has a lot of flavor, so use sparingly!

Nutrient breakdown for the salad per serving and the dressing: Calories: 82, Fat 4 g, (1 g Sat. Fat), Sodium 147 mg, Carbohydrate 10 g, Fiber 4 g, Protein 4 g

Day 20

❏ Limit added sugar:
FIVE grams of added sugar to start with; then 10 g, then 25 g/37 g.

❏ Drink "REAL" water: **FOUR** water bottles, or 64+ ounces every day.

❏ Balanced fuel all day:
THREE balanced meals plus a midday "Strong Snack."

❏ Fill half your plate with non-starchy veggies:
TWO or more non-starchy veggies at lunch and dinner.

❏ Move for 52 minutes!
ONE hour (just about) of make-it-count movement 5 days per week.

❏ Allow a maximum of 25 grams of added sugar for women (that's about 100 calories) and 37 grams for men (about 150 calories).

Have you heard of the 80/20 rule? Some think if you eat well 80% of the time and you will be alright if the other 20% is less than ideal. Be careful with this one. If you don't eat well 20% of the time, you will find these planned splurges collide with the 20% that happens in the unpredictable moments of life, totaling 40%. This could jeopardize the diligent efforts you have put forth 60% of the time.

There is no need to plan to eat unhealthy 20% of the time - life puts us in that position often enough.

Don't go looking for it.

Jay, 49

Has this ever happened to you? For example, you planned for a tasty splurge, and then another one unexpectedly came up right away? Explain:

....

....

123

My recommendation: 100% of the time plan to do what you know is best for you and your family. Only keep foods on hand that promote Your Best Body (at home, work, etc.). Then, when the aforementioned 20% happens without your intentional planning (an unexpected outing, someone bringing your favorite treat by, dinner at a friend's house, or a rushed take-out occasionally on a busy evening), it won't have as great an impact on your health and weight.

Note: if your goal is weight loss, the lower that percentage is, the quicker you will see Best Body results. But, don't be so rigid that you are tempted to give up.

❏ Log your food on My Fitness Pal or a similar electronic tracking program/app today (use a copy of Appendix E if you are unable to enter it directly into an electronic tracking program or app, but be sure to transfer it as soon as you can).

❏ Swap food records with your partner at the end of the day, making a note on your partner's food log regarding what you think I would say about his/her day's intake based on what you have learned so far in this Success Journal.

❏ Look over your day's log and don't let that 20% creep up! If you occasionally have a cookie with lunch, think to yourself: "What a satisfying treat! I am not at all deprived! There is no need for me to go hunting for another indulgence at every opportunity."

Have you been weighing and plotting your weight about once a week on Appendix C's graph?.........Take a look at your graph for a moment. Are you making the progress you were anticipating?

....

....

Brainstorm why or why not:

....

....

....

....

Day 19

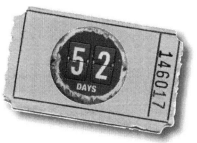

❏ Allow a maximum of 25 grams of added sugar for women (that's about 100 calories) and 37 grams for men (about 150 calories).

❏ Rest from vigorous exercise today, but make sure you are on your feet being active at least 52 minutes of the day.

❏ Limit added sugar:
FIVE grams of added sugar to start with; then 10 g, then 25 g/37 g.

❏ Drink "REAL" water:
FOUR water bottles, or 64+ ounces every day.

❏ Balanced fuel all day:
THREE balanced meals plus a midday "Strong Snack."

❏ Fill half your plate with non-starchy veggies:
TWO or more non-starchy veggies at lunch and dinner.

❏ Move for 52 minutes!
ONE hour (just about) of make-it-count movement 5 days per week.

❏ Rest today, but time your plank; how long can you hold it with good form before you need to stop? ....minutes and .... seconds.

❏ Visualize yourself having achieved the goal(s) you set for this 52 day Countdown. Think about what you will do with your new strength and confidence. What can you do now, or will you be able to do soon, that you could not or would not have done before?

....

....

Exercising most days of the week is part of an active lifestyle. Did you know that some studies show that those who exercise intensely are often sedentary the rest of the day? Should exercisers take the elevator instead of the stairs "because they can?" Is that an active lifestyle? Not really. Don't skip the walk to the mailbox because of your tough workout. If your workout is so fatiguing or produces so much soreness that you feel like you have to sit the rest of the day to recover, then you need to reevaluate.

When I lived on the coast, I would observe my quiet beach as it would get busy over the summer holidays. There were families that all sat together on lounge chairs and passed around the chip bags, only getting up to go to the cooler. And then there were families that threw the frisbee, splashed in the waves, and took walks at low tide. I can't speak for their genes, but I can tell you these families looked different from one another, at least partly because their behavior was different.

Does your family spend most of the time in the kitchen and on the couch, or outside and in motion?

....

Think about what separates the "active" from the 1-hour exercisers. Active people don't circle the parking lot looking for the closest spot, but just enjoy the walk. The children of active people are usually active, too, and not complaining that Mom always has them run upstairs to get something for her, or that Dad never gets up to get the remote himself.

We cannot solve our problems with the same thinking we used when we created them.
Albert Einstein

What can you do to become a more active person in general?

....

....

....

❏   Decide with your accountability partner and friends/family which annual 5Ks or 10Ks you will commit to doing together, or something similar. Check out active.com for ideas, or your local sports council's web calendar. There are so many great causes to support while being active! Which ones interest you during the following seasons?

Winter: ....

Spring:..

Summer:..

Fall:..

Join me and my family annually at the Trot to Adopt 5K/1 mile Family Fun Run Evans, Georgia – TrotToAdopt.org

What kinds of outings or vacations are suited for fit, active people like you? Family bike rides on the weekends? Maybe a hiking or skiing trip? Perhaps you could join a pool, or try something you never would have done before like becoming part of a tennis team, a cycling or running club, or a softball team. Maybe you could try ballroom dancing, or lead an aerobics or cycle class.

❏ Circle any of the above that you are willing to try.

I started teaching aerobics when I was 19, and I have exercised almost every day for 18+ years because of it! Though I am committed to an active lifestyle, I can't promise that I would have been as consistent without this regular commitment. Build accountability into your life to set yourself up for ongoing success!

What activities will you start doing as you reach Your Best Body during the following times?

weekends:..

holidays: ....

vacations: ....

afternoons or evenings: ....

Day 18

❑ Limit added sugar:
FIVE grams of added sugar to start with; then 10 g, then 25 g/37 g.

❑ Drink "REAL" water:
FOUR water bottles, or 64+ ounces every day.

❑ Balanced fuel all day:
THREE balanced meals plus a midday "Strong Snack."

❑ Fill half your plate with non-starchy veggies:
TWO or more non-starchy veggies at lunch and dinner.

❑ Move for 52 minutes!
ONE hour (just about) of make-it-count movement 5 days per week.

❑ Allow a maximum of 25 grams of added sugar for women (that's about 100 calories) and 37 grams for men (about 150 calories).

Which of the following defines a snack? (check)
- ○ anything at all that I eat when it is not meal time
- ○ anything I get from the vending machine
- ○ something that is salty
- ○ something that is sweet
- ○ something that I can eat from a crinkly package
- ○ anything I eat standing up, or on the go

128

○ whatever I can find in a "100-calorie pack"

○ food to hold me from one balanced meal to the next balanced meal without getting too hungry

○ an opportunity to get in some nutrients that I didn't get at my last meal (think: fruit, fiber, calcium or Vitamin D-rich foods, veggies)

You may have guessed where I was heading...the last two are my definitions of a "snack." As you know, I recommend mid-day "Strong Snacks," and an additional mid-morning one when necessary for those with long, active days.

❑ Today, and ideally for the next 18 days and beyond, intentionally avoid having snacks that do not fit the "Strong Snack" profile. Remember, in total, it should have at least 5 grams of protein and 3 grams of fiber to count as a "Strong Snack." If you need a snack to hold you over from breakfast to lunch, please pick a food from one, two or three of the "Strong Snack" columns in the chart on Day 46, depending upon which kind of "car you drive" and "how far you are driving" today. If you are within an hour or two of a meal and feel you must have a snack to hold over, then one fruit serving is often sufficient. Refer to the example of this on the Sample Menu in Appendix K.

Ideally, save your grains for meals instead of snacks, and eat the satisfying "Strong Snack" combination from the table on Day 46. Why, you ask? I have found that having "snack-y" foods like sweetened crackers/grains for snack time often sets people up to overeat, craving more of the same. They are not as filling or as nutritious, either. Though I like the sweetness of an apple, I am happy with just one as part of my "Strong Snack," and I can't always say the same if I have a cookie.

❑ Make up a "Strong Snack" bin or cooler for the next 5 days. If applicable, bring it to work to keep in the refrigerator there for the week, or at home. Then you are set up to successfully avoid the vending machine or the all too often surveying of your pantry's contents.

Day 17

❑ Limit added sugar:
FIVE grams of added sugar to start with;
then 10 g, then 25 g/37 g.

❑ Drink "REAL" water:
FOUR water bottles, or
64+ ounces every day.

❑ Balanced fuel all day:
THREE balanced meals plus a midday "Strong Snack."

❑ Fill half your plate with non-starchy veggies:
TWO or more non-starchy veggies at lunch and dinner.

❑ Move for 52 minutes!
ONE hour (just about) of make-it-count movement 5 days per week.

❑ Allow a maximum of 25 grams of added sugar for women (that's about 100 calories) and 37 grams for men (about 150 calories).

Many people think they are eating healthy when their calories are low, when they are eating organic foods, or when they aren't eating greasy foods or bread. Even if your calories are in the appropriate range for your weight goals, your body desires whole, healthful fuel to operate your metabolism at its best. However, don't be fooled into thinking that "premium fuel" won't spill over into your fat cell stores if you have too much of it. Aim not only for healthy food as fuel, but eat it in the proper amounts considering your activity level so that you do not take in excess, which your body has to store as fat tissue.

Would you do better if you measured everything this week and kept a daily food log? If so, will you?

....

....

❑ Do not eat any processed food all day. Choose instead foods that are much like their original form and that contain just a handful of ingredients at the most. Can you keep this up most of the time? ....This is a life-changer!

130

When I avoid processed food, I feel clean inside and out and don't have migraines, cramps, bloating, or complexion problems.

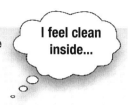

Nicole, 33

If I walked in your home unannounced and flung open the pantry and refrigerator doors right now (don't worry, I probably won't), which would I be more likely to say? (check)

○ "Wow! I see why you have done so well over this Countdown!"

○ "Well, I see what needs to happen here to get you on the right track so you can reach Your Best Body!"

Day 16

5 ❏ Limit added sugar:
FIVE grams of added sugar to start with; then 10 g, then 25 g/37 g.

4 ❏ Drink "REAL" water:
FOUR water bottles, or 64+ ounces every day.

3 ❏ Balanced fuel all day:
THREE balanced meals plus a midday "Strong Snack."

2 ❏ Fill half your plate with non-starchy veggies:
TWO or more non-starchy veggies at lunch and dinner.

1 ❏ Move for 52 minutes!
ONE hour (just about) of make-it-count movement 5 days per week.

❏ Allow a maximum of 25 grams of added sugar for women (that's about 100 calories) and 37 grams for men (about 150 calories).

❏ Rest from vigorous exercise today, but make sure you are on your feet being active at least 52 minutes of the day.

131

❏ Time your plank. How long can you hold it with good form before you need to stop? ....minutes and ....seconds

Do you drink anything else besides water? If you are following the current "Countdown: 5, 4, 3, 2, 1" guidelines, then you are not likely drinking caloric beverages, or they would send you quickly over your sugar limit of 25/37 grams of added sugar per day. Just one can of soda has about 40 grams of added sugar (10 teaspoons). Will you commit to steering clear of any caloric beverages you were having before the Countdown began? ....

What sort of drinks do you like? Make a list below including juice, shakes, alcoholic beverages, sodas, teas, and coffee with whatever you add to it.

....

....

....

❏ Look up the calories for 16 ounces (2 cups) of the beverages noted above online (try caloriecount.com or supertracker.usda.gov) and write the number of calories into the margin to the right of each beverage. It will most likely add up more than you realized!

"Richard Mattes of Purdue University gave 15 normal-weight men and women an extra 450 calories a day as either a liquid (three 12-ounce cans of soda) or solid (45 large jelly beans) for 4 weeks each.
    'When they got the solid food, they ate less at other times, so they adjusted for all of the calories,' he explains. In contrast, 'when they got the liquid food, they just added those calories to their customary diet. They didn't compensate at all.'
    Other studies also suggest that people compensate best for solid foods, less well for semi-solid foods like (non-clear) soup or milkshakes, and worst for liquids, he adds. 'Liquid calories don't trip our satiety mechanisms. They just don't register.' says Mattes."

Permission for use granted by the Center for Science in the Public Interest.

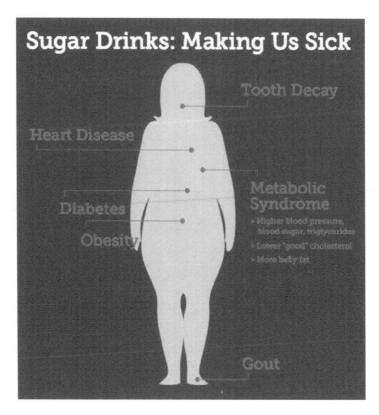

Sugar Drinks: Making Us Sick

Tooth Decay

Heart Disease

Diabetes

Obesity

Metabolic Syndrome
> Higher blood pressure, blood sugar, triglycerides
> Lower "good" cholesterol
> More belly fat

Gout

Milk is a caloric beverage, but its nutritive qualities are much like a food's. Unless sweetened, the sugar in cow's milk occurs naturally as lactose. Though most adults do not, it certainly is possible to exceed your caloric needs with even a health-promoting beverage such as milk, soy milk, rice milk or almond milk.

FAQ

Q: What about diet drinks?

A: Though "diet" drinks are sweetened artificially and do not contain calories, it is still wise to limit these additives to a maximum of one or two artificially sweetened items/day (including gum, yogurts, etc.). Stevia or Splenda/sucralose are the safest.

❏ Peek ahead to Day 13 so you have time to plan some fun...

Day 15

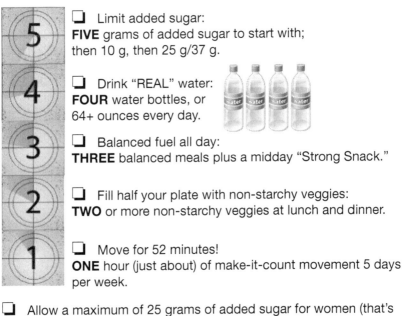

❑ Limit added sugar:
FIVE grams of added sugar to start with; then 10 g, then 25 g/37 g.

❑ Drink "REAL" water:
FOUR water bottles, or 64+ ounces every day.

❑ Balanced fuel all day:
THREE balanced meals plus a midday "Strong Snack."

❑ Fill half your plate with non-starchy veggies:
TWO or more non-starchy veggies at lunch and dinner.

❑ Move for 52 minutes!
ONE hour (just about) of make-it-count movement 5 days per week.

❑ Allow a maximum of 25 grams of added sugar for women (that's about 100 calories) and 37 grams for men (about 150 calories).

❑ Do a "Take Ten" three times today. The following set of 10-minute exercises is the most difficult intensity of the "Take Tens" and is for intermediate-advanced level exercisers. Feel free to use the "Take Tens" from Day 49 or Day 31 if you are not ready for this level, or go ahead and give this one a try at your own pace. Remember to catch your breath briefly as needed as you transition between each minute.

See http://www.acefitness.org/acefit/exercise-library-main/ for proper form if needed, typing the name of the exercise with the asterisk in the search bar.

Take Ten

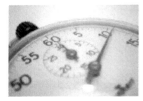

Minute 1: punching bag arms (increasing speed as you warm up), while holding a wide, low squat (toes out) - 30 sec R, 30 sec L
Minute 2: 30-second plank*; (beginners, continue to hold plank; advanced, do squat thrusts/burpees for the second 30 seconds)
Minute 3: sprinter pulls* (aka "screamers") - 10 R, 10 L; repeat until the minute is up

Minute 4: side plank with straight leg* (bent lower leg for beginners) - 30 sec R, 30 sec L
Minute 5: lunge forward R (knee over ankle), step feet together, and lunge back L, step feet together - 30 seconds, then switch lead leg for 30 seconds
Minute 6: 30 sec pushups, 30 sec triceps dips
Minute 7: fast feet (sprint in place) - 30 seconds; wall squat - hold for 30 seconds (back flat against the wall, legs in front as if seated in an imaginary chair, keeping knees over ankles)
Minute 8: explosive jump up on a step or stair, then step down; repeat
Minute 9: hold your balance while doing a side kick with 1 leg with a quick toe tap down before lifting for another side kick - 30 sec R side, 30 sec L; allow yourself an extra moment of slow moving to cool down before finishing with abs in Minute 10
Minute 10: supine bicycle crunches*

Be sure to take a few minutes to cool-down and stretch afterwards. Use the following link if you need a guide for stretching: http://www.mayoclinic.com/health/stretching/SM00043&slide=2

❏ Email or text your partner: "I did Day 15's 'Take Ten' three times today, and it was ....!"

You only have 22 "Don't just stand there, move!" minutes left to complete today! Just move whenever you can!

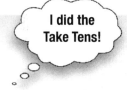

I did the "Take Tens!" We were traveling so I did it first in the morning at the hotel with the kids cheering me on. Then I did the second and third back to back once we arrived to our destination. It wasn't easy, but it feels great to get it done!

Tom, 38

❏ Portion-power check-up! Quickly pick out your favorite cereal from your pantry and pour your typical portion into your everyday bowl (without milk). Then, go back and measure it. Check it against the label's serving size to find the number of carbohydrates your serving amounts to. If you don't eat cereal often, try this with rice or crackers or another carbohydrate you tend to eat regularly.

Fifteen grams of carbohydrate is considered a serving. Unless you are an athlete utilizing lots of fuel, or a growing teen, 1-3 carbohydrate servings (15-45 grams) from grain or starch at each of your 3 meals is appropriate (higher end for those who are very active or have a lot of lean body mass, lower end otherwise).

15-45 g carb from grains, starchy vegetables and beans

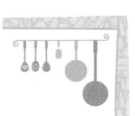

If you are going to occasionally have a dessert, or Mexican, Chinese or Italian food, your carbs will likely surpass that 15-45 grams instantly, so only choose those options if you are brimming with self-control. Or, perhaps you know your limits and find it best to make a different choice all together. By the time your day is wrapping up, often one or two grain/starch servings at dinner is plenty (15-30 g carbs). Visualize a serving the size of your computer mouse - that's about 1/2 cup (equal to roughly 15 grams). Don't forget, Appendix J has serving sizes listed for each food group as a guide; the food servings listed in the columns for grains and starchy vegetables are equal to 15 grams of carbohydrate. When in doubt, check the label to portion your servings into increments of 15 grams of carbohydrate. If a label is not available, go with a 1/2 cup serving.

Pita Chips

Serves 4

2 pitas (whole wheat/oat bran)
2 teaspoons olive oil
1/8 teaspoon of Cavender's Greek seasoning
1/4 teaspoon of Mrs. Dash Garlic and Herb seasoning

Cut or tear whole wheat or oat bran pitas into wedges.
Spray or brush lightly with olive oil and sprinkle with seasoning.
Bake on a cookie sheet at 400 degrees until warm and beginning to brown, about 3-6 minutes.

These are also great to serve with hummus dip.

Nutrient Breakdown: Calories 120, Fat 7 g, Sodium 120 mg, Carbohydrate 12 g, Fiber 2 g, Protein 2 g

Day 14

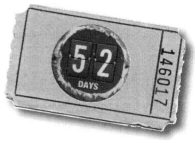

❑ Allow a maximum of 25 grams of added sugar for women (that's about 100 calories) and 37 grams for men (about 150 calories).

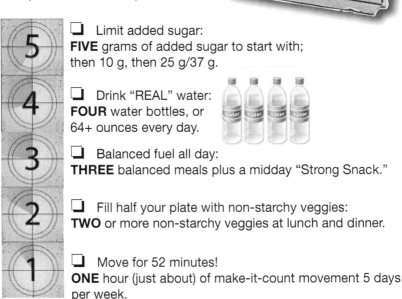

❑ Limit added sugar:
FIVE grams of added sugar to start with; then 10 g, then 25 g/37 g.

❑ Drink "REAL" water:
FOUR water bottles, or 64+ ounces every day.

❑ Balanced fuel all day:
THREE balanced meals plus a midday "Strong Snack."

❑ Fill half your plate with non-starchy veggies:
TWO or more non-starchy veggies at lunch and dinner.

❑ Move for 52 minutes!
ONE hour (just about) of make-it-count movement 5 days per week.

You have just two weeks until your Countdown is complete!
❑ Today, write out a 2-week meal plan for dinners on the following two pages, incorporating some of the meals you used on Day 30's meal planning worksheet, and new or modified options you have tried since then.

❑ Plan to repeat your menu right after you successfully finish this Countdown. You can download the meal planning worksheet from bestbodyin52.com or make copies of it from Appendix G. Add any new favorites to create a 2-3 week rotation of meals to use regularly at home. This will keep things simple and before you know it, your menu planning will be on auto-pilot.

Week 1

MEAL PLANNING	PICTURE IT!	GROCERY NEEDS	PREPARATION TIPS
Monday's Dinner			
Tuesday's Dinner			
Wednesday's Dinner			
Thursday's Dinner			
Friday's Dinner			
Saturday's Dinner			
Sunday's Dinner			

138

Week 2

MEAL PLANNING	PICTURE IT!	GROCERY NEEDS	PREPARATION TIPS
Monday's Dinner			
Tuesday's Dinner			
Wednesday's Dinner			
Thursday's Dinner			
Friday's Dinner			
Saturday's Dinner			
Sunday's Dinner			

Day 13

❏ Limit added sugar:
FIVE grams of added sugar to start with;
then 10 g, then 25 g/37 g.

❏ Drink "REAL" water:
FOUR water bottles, or
64+ ounces every day.

❏ Balanced fuel all day:
THREE balanced meals plus a midday "Strong Snack."

❏ Fill half your plate with non-starchy veggies:
TWO or more non-starchy veggies at lunch and dinner.

❏ Move for 52 minutes!
ONE hour (just about) of make-it-count movement 5 days
per week.

❏ Allow a maximum of 25 grams of added sugar for women (that's
about 100 calories) and 37 grams for men (about 150 calories).

❏ Schedule some recreation time for today with friends and family
(or within the next 3 days if today is not feasible). What can you do
that will keep you moving for at least 52 minutes that makes time fly
by because it is fun? Do you have Wii Fit or an exercise DVD you once
loved? Maybe you could organize a neighborhood kickball or softball
game, or toss the football or frisbee. Try a timed water-treading
contest at a nearby pool or lake, or go for a hike or a canoe ride.

❏ Get adventurous! Go through your calendar and schedule
something every other weekend for the next 6 weeks that is active
play. (See facing page.) Scheduling it with loved ones not only makes
it more fun, but keeps you committed to following through.

Look back to the continuum you marked on Day 40 regarding whole
grains. How is your follow-through on that commitment going?

....

....

UPCOMING ACTIVE FUN EVENT	WITH WHOM?
Today's adventure:	
2 weeks from now (Date: ....)	
4 weeks from now (Date: ....)	
6 weeks from now (Date: ....)	

Day 12

❑ Limit added sugar:
FIVE grams of added sugar to start with; then 10 g, then 25 g/37 g.

❑ Drink "REAL" water:
FOUR water bottles, or 64+ ounces every day.

❑ Balanced fuel all day:
THREE balanced meals plus a midday "Strong Snack."

❑ Fill half your plate with non-starchy veggies:
TWO or more non-starchy veggies at lunch and dinner.

❑ Move for 52 minutes!
ONE hour (just about) of make-it-count movement 5 days per week.

❑ Allow a maximum of 25 grams of added sugar for women (that's about 100 calories) and 37 grams for men (about 150 calories).

❑ Rest from vigorous exercise today, but make sure you are on your feet being active at least 52 minutes of the day.

❏   Time your plank. How long can you hold it with good form before you need to stop? ....minutes and ....seconds

Is there such a thing as a "safe splurge?" If chocolate is your very greatest temptation, and most favorite food, which of these would be a "safe splurge"?

a) Buy a bag of Hershey's kisses on sale after Halloween, but keep them in the freezer for a time of need.

b) When you make cookies at home, try to get your friends and family to eat them all so you don't get stuck having to face them.

c) When you buy your kids snacks for a special event at school, get only the single servings and no extras. That's just one for each of them, and one for you (if it's really worth it).

d) Get the sale 8-pack of snack size candy bars and eat them all at once so you don't have to longingly gaze at them anymore.

e) Call your accountability partner and suggest celebrating your progress with a brownie a la mode at a nearby restaurant.

The answer is C, of course. Set yourself up for success! Only eat your most tempting foods in controlled settings (and ideally with another adult who will hold you accountable). Remember, a splurge is most enjoyable when you savor each bite intentionally. A safe splurge is not a whole week of "all you can eat indulgence" on a cruise, for example. Even when having a special dinner, such as on your Anniversary, instead of splurging on the appetizer, a glass of wine or two, your favorite creamy entree, and dessert, splurge on just one or two of those and savor every bite or sip, only finishing what you really want.

Note your most tempting food(s) in the corresponding lines below.

I have done well with the following temptations:

....

....

I'm still struggling with these:

....

....

From now on, I will only eat my most tempting foods in a controlled "safe splurge" setting such as:

....

....

No more eating Oreos with my three year-old. I am just not going to buy them.

Anonymous, 29

No more eating Oreos with my 3-year-old.

Day 11

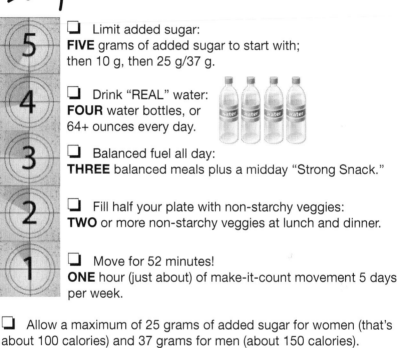

❑ Limit added sugar:
FIVE grams of added sugar to start with; then 10 g, then 25 g/37 g.

❑ Drink "REAL" water:
FOUR water bottles, or 64+ ounces every day.

❑ Balanced fuel all day:
THREE balanced meals plus a midday "Strong Snack."

❑ Fill half your plate with non-starchy veggies:
TWO or more non-starchy veggies at lunch and dinner.

❑ Move for 52 minutes!
ONE hour (just about) of make-it-count movement 5 days per week.

❑ Allow a maximum of 25 grams of added sugar for women (that's about 100 calories) and 37 grams for men (about 150 calories).

❑ Log your food on My Fitness Pal or a similar electronic tracking program/app today (use a copy of Appendix E if needed).

You are on the home stretch! Less than two weeks to go to reach Your Best Body! My intention with this publication is not just to help you see results at the 52 day mark, but also to set you up for "healthfully ever after!"

Imagine...soon enough you'll have the labels of your favorite healthy foods memorized...a rotating menu plan that you can shop for with your eyes closed...you might find yourself kayaking on weekends...breathing easy after three flights of stairs...spending your fast food money on a new bike or a hiking trip...cooking a healthy dinner for friends instead of meeting out for burgers and fries...clothes shopping in the section of the store you have always wanted to find yourself in...enjoying foods you always said you hated...you might even be accused of being one of those "naturally thin" people.

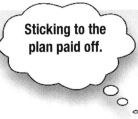

Sticking to the plan paid off.

The strategies and encouragement of the Countdown were life changing to me! Sticking to the plan paid off: self-control challenged, weight lost, new habits in place, and confidence built!

Karla, 38

Visualize yourself at your goal. Picture how you will look and imagine how you will feel. What words or phrases will describe your outlook on life and your healthful future? How will others describe you?

List five to ten phrases that will best describe you once you have reached your goal:

1. ....
2. ....
3. ....
4. ....
5. ....
6. ....
7. ....
8. ....
9. ....
10. ....

Day 10

5 ❏ Limit added sugar:
FIVE grams of added sugar to start with;
then 10 g, then 25 g/37 g.

4 ❏ Drink "REAL" water:
FOUR water bottles, or
64+ ounces every day.

3 ❏ Balanced fuel all day:
THREE balanced meals plus a midday "Strong Snack."

2 ❏ Fill half your plate with non-starchy veggies:
TWO or more non-starchy veggies at lunch and dinner.

1 ❏ Move for 52 minutes!
ONE hour (just about) of make-it-count movement 5 days
per week.

❏ Allow a maximum of 25 grams of added sugar for women (that's about 100 calories) and 37 grams for men (about 150 calories).

❏ If it will pump you up for the big finish, sing one of the following at the very top of your lungs: "The Final Countdown," "Eye of the Tiger," or "Gonna Fly Now." Just 10 days until you are there!

❏ Make a playlist or CD for these next several days of exercise so that you'll be crossing the finish line with your most motivating tunes in the background. You must take intentional steps to make your active lifestyle enjoyable or you will end up on the couch.

❏ Make an exercise plan with your partner and write it on your calendar (or put it into your electronic calendar) for the next 10 days. Plan a workout this week that is different than anything you've done over the course of this Countdown. Mark off each day on your calendar once it is complete.

What have you learned from this Countdown so far that you didn't know before, that you believe will stick with you?

....

....

❑ To keep learning, sign up for the Daily Tip emails by *Nutrition Action Healthletter*. It's a free resource that is easy, enjoyable reading and will keep you making great food choices year-round: nutritionaction.com.

Roasted Asparagus with Garlic and Lemon

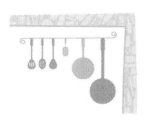

Serves 4

1 pound of fresh asparagus
1 teaspoon olive oil
1/8 teaspoon black pepper
1/8 teaspoon salt
1 tablespoon lemon juice (or juice from _ lemon)
1 clove garlic, minced
2 tablespoon pine nuts, toasted (optional but delicious)
Vegetable oil cooking spray

1. Preheat oven to 400 degrees.
2. Cover a baking sheet with aluminum foil (for easy clean up) and spray with vegetable oil cooking spray. Snap the tough/woody ends off each asparagus spear and discard. Cut asparagus into large bite size pieces and place in a large bowl. Add the olive oil, pepper, salt, lemon juice, and garlic. Toss to coat.
3. Transfer asparagus to the baking sheet and roast for 7-9 minutes until tender and slightly brown. Stir halfway through cooking time.
4. Meanwhile, toast the pine nuts in a dry skillet over medium heat for 3-4 minutes, stirring occasionally until they are fragrant and brown.
5. To serve, transfer asparagus to a serving platter and sprinkle with toasted nuts.

Nutrient breakdown: Calories 70, Fat 4 g, Carb 6 g, Fiber 3 g, Protein 3 g (without the nuts this recipe has 40 calories, and 1 g of fat)
Recipe contributed by Kim Beavers, MS, RD, LD, CDE

Day 9

❏ Limit added sugar:
FIVE grams of added sugar to start with; then 10 g, then 25 g/37 g.

❏ Drink "REAL" water:
FOUR water bottles, or 64+ ounces every day.

❏ Balanced fuel all day:
THREE balanced meals plus a midday "Strong Snack."

❏ Fill half your plate with non-starchy veggies:
TWO or more non-starchy veggies at lunch and dinner.

❏ Move for 52 minutes!
ONE hour (just about) of make-it-count movement 5 days per week.

❏ Allow a maximum of 25 grams of added sugar for women (that's about 100 calories) and 37 grams for men (about 150 calories).

❏ Rest from vigorous exercise today, but make sure you are on your feet being active at least 52 minutes of the day.

❏ Time your plank. How long can you hold it with good form before you need to stop? ....minutes and ....seconds

What are the two main anchors that have kept you in this 52 day Countdown all the way to this point? Only the SUPER-STRONG make it this far! You should be proud of yourself!

....

....

What behavior change have you made over these last 43 days that you are most pleased with yourself for maintaining?

....

....

Below, list the pros and cons for maintaining your healthy, active lifestyle beyond these final days of the Countdown (or even for starting it again if you have a bit to go still).

PROS	CONS
....	....
....	....
....	....

Day 8

❏ Limit added sugar:
FIVE grams of added sugar to start with; then 10 g, then 25 g/37 g.

❏ Drink "REAL" water:
FOUR water bottles, or 64+ ounces every day.

❏ Balanced fuel all day:
THREE balanced meals plus a midday "Strong Snack."

❏ Fill half your plate with non-starchy veggies:
TWO or more non-starchy veggies at lunch and dinner.

❏ Move for 52 minutes!
ONE hour (just about) of make-it-count movement 5 days per week.

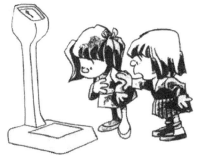

"Don't step on it! It makes you cry!

❏ Allow a maximum of 25 grams of added sugar for women (that's about 100 calories) and 37 grams for men (about 150 calories).

Does using a scale motivate you? .... How often do you weigh yourself? .... Weighing keeps some people in check and whenever they hit a certain point,

148

they fly straighter. For others who get discouraged by fluctuations, it sets a poor tone for their day rather than propelling change. According to the National Weight Control Registry, maintaining the accountability provided by weighing weekly is key to the success of 75% of those who have kept their weight off for over five years.

Have you been plotting your weight on Appendix C's graph?.............
Does it help you to see your weekly weight trend on the graph?............

❏ If your scale does more harm than good for your overall health goals, then take it to the thrift shop. You can weigh elsewhere if you still want to record your weekly weight, or instead, track measurements.

❏ Most people can tell by how their clothes fit if their weight is going up or down. If your clothes are so baggy and stretchy that you can't tell when you are gaining weight, it is time to put on a belt. I have heard clients say they regret wearing stretchy clothes over the holidays because that material did not help with accountability. It is so much harder to take off the average 4-6 holiday pounds than it is to put them on!

❏ Mark your calendar to set yourself up the following Holiday challenges for the upcoming year. (Check below once you have added each to your calendar).
◯ New Year's Day: Review your Success Journal annually for a reminder of what works well for you and to be prepared for any barriers and challenges.
◯ Valentine's Day: Enjoy one reasonable piece of a Valentine's treat very slowly and mindfully, taking small bites.
◯ Easter: Decide how you want to spend a 200 calorie splurge and stop there.
◯ Summer holidays: Write out a plan for exactly what you'll eat and drink before your celebration for each of the following holidays, and stick to your plan.
   ◯ Memorial Day
   ◯ July 4th
   ◯ Labor Day
◯ Halloween: No candy on Halloween. Or for a greater challenge, try going without candy the entire week of Halloween. You'll gain confidence in your will power!

○ Thanksgiving: Do 10 "Take Tens" over the course of the 7-day week.

○ Christmas: Write down every bite and sip that you have on the 24th, 25th, and 26th of December.

❏ I have seen many people fall off track when a holiday gets them out of routine. Enlist your partner to take on the holiday challenges with you year-round. Is he/she in? ....

What are you planning to do for accountability when this Countdown is complete in just one week?

....

....

Day 7

❏ Limit added sugar: **FIVE** grams of added sugar to start with; then 10 g, then 25 g/37 g.

❏ Drink "REAL" water: **FOUR** water bottles, or 64+ ounces every day.

❏ Balanced fuel all day: **THREE** balanced meals plus a midday "Strong Snack."

❏ Fill half your plate with non-starchy veggies: **TWO** or more non-starchy veggies at lunch and dinner.

❏ Move for 52 minutes! **ONE** hour (just about) of make-it-count movement 5 days per week.

❏ Allow a maximum of 25 grams of added sugar for women (that's about 100 calories) and 37 grams for men (about 150 calories).

If you ate more slowly, would you perhaps be satisfied with less? Fast eaters typically eat more than they would if they were eating slowly.

Researchers told 30 young normal-weight women to eat as much at lunch as they wanted, either quickly or slowly. The quick meals lasted about 9 minutes. The women consumed 65 fewer calories at the slow meals, which averaged about 29 minutes. That may not seem like a lot of calories, but over 3 meals daily, it certainly adds up...remember 100 extra calories daily equals about 10 pounds of fat tissue annually.

Most men pursue pleasure with such breathless haste that they hurry past it.

Soren Kierkegaard

❏ At all of your meals today, try these three tips to slow your meal down.
　1) use a smaller spoon or fork than you typically do
　2) take small bites, putting the utensil down between bites
　3) chew each bite many times before swallowing

❏ Log your food on My Fitness Pal or a similar electronic tracking program/app today (use a copy of Appendix E if needed).

❏ Print out your food log at the end of the day and grade it with a red pen as if you were a teacher. What could you improve to reach Your Best Body?

....

....

Can you tell a difference in your body fat? For example, does it feel different across your middle when you buckle in your seatbelt? Are you more comfortable in your clothes?

....

....

❏ Be sure to check out INDESTRUCTIBLE at bestbodyin52.com for ongoing accountability, meal plans, recipes, and many more success strategies I have put together to keep you at your best.

Day 6

❏ Limit added sugar:
FIVE grams of added sugar to start with; then 10 g, then 25 g/37 g.

❏ Drink "REAL" water:
FOUR water bottles, or 64+ ounces every day.

❏ Balanced fuel all day:
THREE balanced meals plus a midday "Strong Snack."

❏ Fill half your plate with non-starchy veggies:
TWO or more non-starchy veggies at lunch and dinner.

❏ Move for 52 minutes!
ONE hour (just about) of make-it-count movement 5 days per week.

❏ Allow a maximum of 25 grams of added sugar for women (that's about 100 calories) and 37 grams for men (about 150 calories).

It takes about 6 weeks to form a new habit, and you have reached that point! Without looking, see if you can recall from memory the five foundational strategies of this program (hint: "Countdown 5, 4, 3, 2, 1"). Do any of these five feel like second nature to you now? Why or why not?

....

....

....

❏ Highlight any of the five foundational strategies above that are not quite routine for you yet.

List two new habits you have formed of which you are proud:

....

....

152

Which old habits do you pledge to never go back to?

....

....

Which habits could get you into trouble if you are not cautious?

....

....

❏   Email or text your accountability partner the habits you pledge to never revisit.

Southwestern Chopped Salad

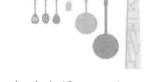

Serves 4 (as a complete meal)

1-1/4 pounds sirloin steak
2 tablespoons Mrs. Dash Chipotle Seasoning
1/2 tablespoon olive oil
Taylor Farms, Dole, or other Southwest Chopped salad, 10-ounce bag
1/2 cup reduced fat (or 2%) cheddar cheese, shredded
1 can reduced-sodium black beans, rinsed and drained

1. Cut lean steak into thin strips and place in a zipper seal plastic bag with Mrs. Dash Chipotle Seasoning and olive oil. Let most of the air out of the bag while zipping it. Knead it gently so that the marinade covers the meat. Allow to marinate in the refrigerator for 2 hours, or overnight if possible.
2. To a large bowl filled with the chopped salad ingredients except the dressing, add the cheese and the black beans.
3. Use about 2/3 the dressing packet provided on the entire salad, and toss. I suggest not using the entire packet of dressing from in the salad bag - it's typically high in fat and calories. Or, you could use a separate reduced-fat Southwest-style dressing if desired.
4. Pan-saute the beef (the pan shouldn't need oil because it's in the marinade), leaving a little pink in the center.
5. Serve warm or cold over the salad.

Nutrient Breakdown (includes all of dressing packet): Calories 509, Fat 30 g, Carb 31 g, Sodium 361 mg, Protein 37 g

Day 5

❏ Limit added sugar:
FIVE grams of added sugar to start with; then 10 g, then 25 g/37 g.

❏ Drink "REAL" water:
FOUR water bottles, or 64+ ounces every day.

❏ Balanced fuel all day:
THREE balanced meals plus a midday "Strong Snack."

❏ Fill half your plate with non-starchy veggies:
TWO or more non-starchy veggies at lunch and dinner.

❏ Move for 52 minutes!
ONE hour (just about) of make-it-count movement 5 days per week.

❏ Allow a maximum of 25 grams of added sugar for women (that's about 100 calories) and 37 grams for men (about 150 calories).

❏ Rest from vigorous exercise today, but make sure you are on your feet being active at least 52 minutes of the day.

❏ Time your plank. How long can you hold it with good form before you need to stop? ....minutes and ....seconds.

❏ Stress works against your Best Body progress. Three times today, do any of the following for at least 5 minutes (set a timer if needed): stretch, quiet prayer/meditation time alone and away from distraction, deep breathing exercises, soak in a bubble bath, journal what you are thankful for, or listen to soft music by candlelight. Circle any of the healthy wind-downs you enjoy. Which ones did you do today?

....

....

....

154

What three changes can you make in your life to limit the stress that may be stunting your progress towards Your Best Body?

1. ....
2. ....
3. ....

It's time for a quick quiz over what you have learned during the Countdown to Your Best Body.

1) What type of food should make up the bulk of your plate at lunch and supper?

....

2) What percentage of your day's calories should you consume by 5:00 pm?

....

3) Name two lean cuts of red meat.

....

4) How many times/week should you do strength or resistance training for all major muscle groups?

....

5) What are three foods rich in soluble fiber?

....

6) Name one holiday on which you plan to do the Holiday Challenge, and describe the challenge from memory.

....

7) How many grams of carbohydrate is considered a serving and what is the typical portion size?

....

8) Name two sources of omega-3 fatty acids.

....

9) What are two benefits of drinking 64+ ounces of water daily?

....

10) Give an example of a "Strong Snack."

....

❏ Look up the answers in the Success Journal to confirm yours are correct. That's right, there is not an answer key. Now is a great time for a review!

Day 4

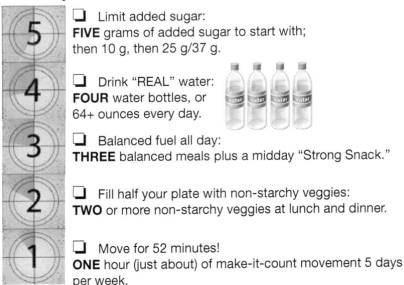

❑ Limit added sugar:
FIVE grams of added sugar to start with; then 10 g, then 25 g/37 g.

❑ Drink "REAL" water:
FOUR water bottles, or 64+ ounces every day.

❑ Balanced fuel all day:
THREE balanced meals plus a midday "Strong Snack."

❑ Fill half your plate with non-starchy veggies:
TWO or more non-starchy veggies at lunch and dinner.

❑ Move for 52 minutes!
ONE hour (just about) of make-it-count movement 5 days per week.

❑ Allow a maximum of 25 grams of added sugar for women (that's about 100 calories) and 37 grams for men (about 150 calories).

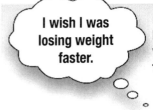

I wish I was losing weight faster.

It's nice that the numbers on the scale keep going down a pound every couple weeks, but I'd really like to lose weight faster.

Laura, 31

Laura has been having steady, slow weight loss progress. She has consistently been exercising 3 times per week, but was not willing to take on an additional workout day or two until she got frustrated with her slow weight loss. After a couple months of doing great with her nutrition, she decided to see what would happen if she put forth her best effort and her time! She couldn't believe how it really did double the speed of her weight loss to fully commit to both my nutrition and exercise recommendations.

> *Whether you think you can or think you can't, you are right.*
> *Henry Ford*

My aerobics class participants can tell you that when we are wrapping up a strenuous piece of an exercise, I often say "let's do four more" and then after those four, I say "four more." Honestly, they can usually do even four more with a little push, though they would not have thought so until they gave it their best effort (along with some encouragement).

What is a challenge or barrier in the way of your success that you know you could conquer if you gave it your very best effort?

....

....

Using the continuum below, what is the likelihood that you will conquer it? (Considering that you have made it just about to the end of the Countdown, I trust you have what it takes!)

I doubt it.   I will do it!

FAQ

Q: Can I shorten my exercise time when the Countdown is complete?

A: If you do not need to lose weight, then 30 minutes of moderate exercise on most days of the week is perfect for health and weight maintenance. But remember, to get rid of those stubborn pounds, it may take exercising 30-90 minutes most days of the week, according to the American College of Sports Medicine. The more fit you become, the more you can push yourself physically and burn calories in less time. In addition to your moderate to intense exercise ("Move it! Move it!"), your body will thank you if you keep up your new "Don't just stand there, move!" habits.

Day 3

5 ☐ Limit added sugar:
FIVE grams of added sugar to start with; then 10 g, then 25 g/37 g.

4 ☐ Drink "REAL" water:
FOUR water bottles, or 64+ ounces every day.

3 ☐ Balanced fuel all day:
THREE balanced meals plus a midday "Strong Snack."

2 ☐ Fill half your plate with non-starchy veggies:
TWO or more non-starchy veggies at lunch and dinner.

1 ☐ Move for 52 minutes!
ONE hour (just about) of make-it-count movement 5 days per week.

☐ Allow a maximum of 25 grams of added sugar for women (that's about 100 calories) and 37 grams for men (about 150 calories).

I have learned from this Countdown that three critical things that I simply must continue long term for my Best Body's sake are:

1. ....

2. ....

3. ....

☐ Write these essential steps to success on three index cards to post at home, in your car, and at work. (Show these for your Ticket.)

☐ Speaking of three...do a "Take Ten" three times today. Since you have three variations to pick from, go ahead and do one of each of them today. They are listed all together in Appendix I for your convenience. Be sure to take time to cool down and stretch after you exercise. Now you have an exercise library to draw from anytime!

❑ Email or text your partner: "I did Day 3's 'Take Ten' three times today, and it was ....!"

❑ Mark your calendar to do a set of "Take Tens" at least once a week for the next 6 weeks.

Take Ten

Day 2

5

❑ Limit added sugar:
FIVE grams of added sugar to start with; then 10 g, then 25 g/37 g.

4

❑ Drink "REAL" water:
FOUR water bottles, or 64+ ounces every day.

3

❑ Balanced fuel all day::
THREE balanced meals plus a midday "Strong Snack."

2

❑ Fill half your plate with non-starchy veggies:
TWO or more non-starchy veggies at lunch and dinner.

1

❑ Move for 52 minutes!
ONE hour (just about) of make-it-count movement 5 days per week.

❑ Allow a maximum of 25 grams of added sugar for women (that's about 100 calories) and 37 grams for men (about 150 calories).

❑ Rest from vigorous exercise today, but make sure you are on your feet being active at least 52 minutes of the day.

❑ Time your plank: .... Look back to your first plank time from the start-up assessment (............), your halfway point plank time (Day 23: ....), and today's plank time (............). How do they compare? ....

Have you been committed to doing the plank exercise twice a week as suggested over the Countdown?............. If so, what benefits have you gained from having this improved core strength?

....

....

> *Without continual growth and progress, such words as improvement, achievement, and success have no meaning.*
>
> Benjamin Franklin

❏   Call or visit your partner and also a good friend and tell them your most impactful VICTORIES from the Countdown to Your Best Body so they can celebrate your progress with you today! Talk with your accountability partner about your next steps. Be thinking about the rewards you planned for yourself - not that any reward could outshine the satisfaction of reaching Your Best Body!

My most impactful victories:

....

....

....

....

My friend said:

....

....

....

....

My accountability partner said:

....

....

....

Talk about the quote by Benjamin Franklin with your accountability parter. Brainstorm together how you'll keep each other accountable in the future for "continual growth and progress." Write it below.

....

....

....

....

You are eligible for the final Best Body ticket if you have filled out the exercise chart weekly (Appendix D).

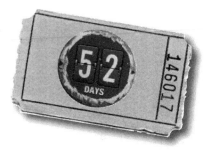

In the space below, make a quick sketch of how you see yourself now that you have completed the Countdown, circling the parts of you that you know have changed for the better.

Drum roll please!

Day 1 (Applause!)

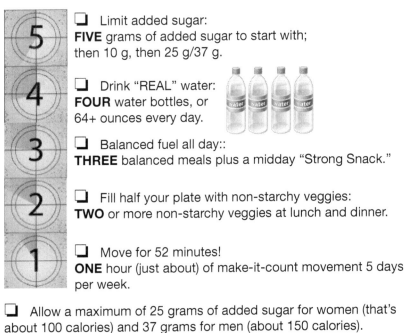

❏ Limit added sugar:
FIVE grams of added sugar to start with; then 10 g, then 25 g/37 g.

❏ Drink "REAL" water:
FOUR water bottles, or 64+ ounces every day.

❏ Balanced fuel all day::
THREE balanced meals plus a midday "Strong Snack."

❏ Fill half your plate with non-starchy veggies:
TWO or more non-starchy veggies at lunch and dinner.

❏ Move for 52 minutes!
ONE hour (just about) of make-it-count movement 5 days per week.

❏ Allow a maximum of 25 grams of added sugar for women (that's about 100 calories) and 37 grams for men (about 150 calories).

Your Best Body!

You made it through the Countdown -
Staying focused for 52 days!
You reached Your Best Body!
You should be proud and amazed -

Astounded by your own progress,
Your leanness and self-control.
You put your health before your urges,
And you have met your goals!

Would you say the prize is worth the price,
Now that you see and feel your success?
Remember "Countdown 5, 4, 3, 2, 1"
So that Your Body stays at its BEST!

You should be very proud of yourself for completing the Success Journal and staying committed, even if you still have a ways to go to reach Your Best Body! **Congratulations on your completion of the 52 day Countdown to Your Best Body!**

❑ Take a picture of the new you and affix it in the front of this journal. Compare it with your other two photos along this journey. Remember, there are even more benefits from the changes on the inside that a picture could never capture.

List 52 things you love about Your Best Body, inside and out! *If you have a long term goal that will take more time, include some that are still in progress. Take a few days off to find a new accountability partner, and then start again strong! Stick with it! You will reach Your Best Body!* Your foundation for success has been set!

1-..
2-..
3-..
4-..
5-..
6-..
7-..
8-..
9-..
10-..
11-..
12-..
13-..
14-..
15-..
16-..
17-..
18-..
19-..
20-..

21-..

22-..

23-..

24-..

25-..

26-..

27-..

28-..

29-..

30-..

31-..

32-..

33-..

34-..

35-..

36-..

37-..

38-..

39-..

40-..

41-..

42-..

43-..

44-..

45-..

46-..

47-..

48-..

49-..

50-..

51-..

52-..

I would love to hear about how you finished strong, and how you feel about Your Best Body. Please keep in touch with me via bestbodyin52.com. Enjoy your "healthfully ever after."

Complete your final progress assessments below and compare them to your initial self assessment.

Date: ....

On a scale of 1-5, (1 being "not at all," and 5 being "definitely"), how did you do on your commitments to the following over the past 52 days?

Completed each day's challenges and filled in answers to the questions.	Stayed committed to my partner/this program for 52 days.	Exercised for 52 minutes, 5 days a week (about half of which was intense).
1 - 2 - 3 - 4 - 5	1 - 2 - 3 - 4 - 5	1 - 2 - 3 - 4 - 5

Never lose an opportunity of seeing anything beautiful. for beauty is God's handwriting.

Ralph Waldo Emerson

After the 52 day Countdown

Name: Date:

Accountability Partner:

Weight: Height:

Waist circumference measurement:......................... inches
Place a cloth tape measure around the smallest part of the waist while standing relaxed.

Measurement in 1 other location where you tend to put on weight/ fat (where exactly: ....and inches:...........................)

Maximum number of seconds you can hold a plank with good form (assessed by someone else): ....minutes..............seconds

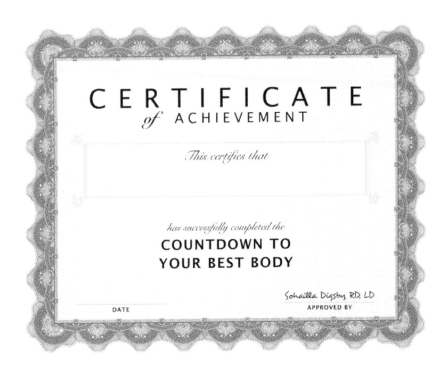

Sources: Selected Resources and References

Academy of Nutrition and Dietetics
American College of Sports Medicine
American Council on Exercise
American Diabetes Association
American Heart Association
Celiac Central
Center for Science in the Public Interest
Mayo Clinic

MedlinePlus, National Library of Medicine
Nancy Clark, RD, LD
National Institutes of Health
Nutrition Action Healthletter
Precise Portions
Sports, Cardiovascular, and Wellness Nutrition Dietetic Practice Group
USDA Choose My Plate

References

Nieman, David C., Weidner, Tom, and Dick, Elliott. "ACSM Current Comment." pages 1-3. Web. December 2013.

Nadelen, Mary D. "Basic Injury Prevention Concepts." ACSM Access Public Information Articles. Jan 10, 2012. page 1. Web. December 2013.

Day 51

Hurley, J. and Liebman, B. "Going Greek. Yogurt Gets a Makeover." Nutrition Action Sept. 2013. pages 13-15.

Day 49

Millar, L.A. ACSM Information on Sprains, Strains, and Tears. American College of Sports Medicine. 2011. pages 1-2. Web. December 2013.

Day 47

Liebman, Bonnie. "Unexpected: Surprising Findings from the Last 40 Years. " Nutrition Action Healthletter. Jan/Feb 2011: 5. Print.

Schardt, David. "Sleep On It: When Counting Sheep Isn't Enough." Nutrition Action Healthletter (2012). Web. 28 October 2013.

Markwald RR, Melanson EL, Smith MR, Higgins J, Perreault L, et al. (2013) "Impact of insufficient sleep on total daily energy expenditure, food intake, and weight gain." Proc Natl Acad Sci USA 110: 5695–5700. Web 28 October 2013.

Shlisky JD, Hartman TJ, Kris–Etherton PM, Rogers CJ, Sharkey NA, Nikols-Richardson SM. "Partial sleep deprivation and energy balance in adults: An emerging issue for consideration by dietetics practitioners." Journal of Academy Nutrition Dietetics. 2012; 112: 1785 – 179. Web 28 October 2013

Day 45

Clark, Nancy. 2003. Nancy Clark's Sports Nutrition Guidebook. Champaign, IL: Human Kinetics.

Office of Dietary Supplements, National Institutes of Health. "Dietary Supplement Fact Sheet: Vitamin B12." 24 June 2011. Web. November 2013.

American Heart Association. "Cooking for Lower Cholesterol." 6 September 2013. Web. December 2013.

Day 44

ACSM Blog writers. (2103, April 29). "Keeping Up with Cooling Down." (Web blog post). Retrieved December 2013 from http://certification.acsm. org/blog/2013/april/keeping-up-with-cooling-down.

Day 41

Liebman, Bonnie and Hurley, Jayne. 2011. Healthy Foods: Your Guide to the Best Basic Foods. Nutrition Action Healthletter. Washington, DC: Center for Science in the Public Interest.

Executive Summary: (2013) "EWG's 2013 Shopper's Guide to Pesticides in Produce." Web. December 2013.

Day 40

National Foundation for Celiac Awareness authors. "Getting Started: Celiac Disease and The Gluten-Free Diet." 2010. Web. September 2013.

American Heart Association. "Whole Grains and Fiber." 24 January 2011. Web. December 2013.

Day 38

Mayo Clinic Staff writers. "Chart of High-Fiber Foods." 2012. Web. November 2013.

Day 32

Wootan, Margo G. and Vickroy, Lindsay. "Informed Eating: Calorie Labeling for Ready_to_Eat Food at Supermarkets and Convenience Stores." November 2012. Web. November 2013.

Day 31

Single-leg dead lift image provided by FitnessforGolf.com

Day 22

Am. J. Clin. Nutr. DOI:10.3945/ajcn.112.039750.

Day 21

Office of Dietary Supplements, National Institutes of Health. "Dietary Supplement Fact Sheet: Calcium." Web. November 2013.

American Heart Association. "Frequently Asked Questions about Better Fats." 6 May 2013. Web. December 2013.

Medline Plus authors. "Vitamin D." 17 May 2012. Web. December 2013.

Day 19

Thompson, Med Sci Sports Exerc 27:347, 1995

FASEB Journal 13: A870, 1999.

Day 16

Am. J. Clin. Nutr. 89: 1299, 2009

Day 7

Am. Diet. Assoc. 108: 1186, 2008.

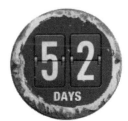

Appendix A

Doing the Countdown to Your Best Body with a Group

Make the most of the Countdown with:
- ○ your coworkers or worksite wellness group
- ○ local gym members
- ○ your singles group
- ○ your local Mom's Club, preschool classroom moms or PTO
- ○ your sports team or your kids' team parents
- ○ your supper club
- ○ your church during a church-wide health stewardship campaign
- ○ your Sunday School class, Small Group, or Bible Study group
- ○ a group of your family and friends

4 Steps to Success

1. Look through your calendar for a good time to run this program for 52 consecutive days with your group. You'll need a couple of weeks to get the Success Journals ordered. Below are some suggestions to consider for starting dates:
- ❏ mid-January, making the most of the start of a New Year
- ❏ 8 weeks prior to your local Spring Break
- ❏ two weeks after Spring Break
- ❏ two weeks after school starts in the fall
- ❏ anytime your prospective group members are interested in weight loss or getting healthy

2. Begin taking registrations and payment for the Success Journal as soon as you start advertising your program so that you can order your books. There is a step-by-step promotional guide in this Appendix.

3. Order your books from bestbodyin52.com if greater than 10 (or via Amazon.com if less than 10). Hold a "Countdown Kick-Off" the week before the 52-day Countdown begins, with plans in place to begin Day 52's challenges on the following Tuesday. At the Countdown Kick-Off:

- ❏ take final registrations (download registration form online)

168

- ❏ give participants their Success Journals and take payment
- ❏ get T-shirt sizes and payment if T-shirts are desired*
- ❏ do fitness assessments
- ❏ do weight/measurements
- ❏ take "before photos"

4. If you start on a Tuesday, the program will end on a Thursday, 52 days later. Plan a simple wrap-up one or two days after the Countdown is complete (that Friday or Saturday, depending on the availability of your participants)
- ❏ do final assessments to assess progress
- ❏ take "after photos"
- ❏ optional: host a healthy potluck/recipe swap and awards ceremony called the "Countdown Completion"

Support
There are varying levels of support and accountability that you, as the coordinator of your Countdown, can provide to increase success. Read on for my suggestions, all of which offer touchpoints and encourage retention.

Camaraderie
- ❏ Create a Facebook "Group" for those who are participating where they can encourage each other, post their before and after photos, and post photos of their balanced plate at meals.
- ❏ *If you would like to order T-shirts (25 minimum per order), please get sizes and payment from participants upon registration. To order, contact me via bestbodyin52.com.
- ❏ Be sure to schedule a group photo with everyone in their T-shirts. Midway through the program is a great time for this!

Opportunity
- ❏ Arrange for a weekly get-together where people can share their successes and barriers to completing the week's Countdown challenges. This is also a good place to offer a weekly weigh-in. (Weight charts can be downloaded from bestbodyin52.com). Ideally, set this up when participants can be active together as a group. Suggestions include a weekly run/walk, hike, group exercise class or DVD, or Boot Camp.
- ❏ If you already have a class scheduled, meet 15 minutes early for a brief time of discussion regarding the Countdown challenges from that week.

❏   Consider hosting a yoga/stretch class (live or via DVD) on the scheduled rest days. If you start on a Tuesday, rest days will fall on Wednesdays and Sundays.

❏   Encourage all participants to sign up for a local 5K to do together during the 52 days.

❏   Decide with the help of the "Winners" guide below if/how you want to reward the "Winners."

Accountability

❏   Have a location where they can "turn in" to you the following 10 "Best Body Ticket Challenges" (or they can post these on your Facebook page to inspire others). As the coordinator of the Countdown, you can either collect all of the following "Best Body Ticket Challenges," or just pick 3-5 of these that are varied and well-spaced over the 52 days.

Place a ticket with the participant's name for each of the following tasks he/she completes into a box or jar for a drawing at the end of the Countdown. Remind them that they must have their names on these documents and on the ticket.

Best Body Ticket Challenges

1) Day 48, 47, and 46's printed food log with name at the top (turn in all 3 days' food records on Day 45)

2) Day 42's journaled self assessment (make a copy or post photographed text)

3) Day 34's printed food log with name written at the top

4) Day 28's Hunger Log

5) Day 23's questions answered as to which strategies they credit

6) Day 19's questions answered about a "new you"

7) Day 14's two-week meal plan

8) Day 7's printed food log with name written at the top

9) Day 3's index cards (a copy or photo of the 3 cards)

10) Exercise check-off chart from the entire program (Appendix D)

"Winners"

All who stick with the Countdown for 52 days should be applauded. If you decide you want to have an incentive for those who do especially well in this challenge, please find my recommendations below.

The assessment to determine who wins should not be based primarily on weight loss. Keep in mind that not everyone working to achieve their Best Body needs to lose weight (for instance, some want to gain muscle, or change their eating habits, but to maintain their weight). I suggest that a "ticket" is put in a "hat" for each of those above (1-10) once turned in to you or posted. (See website for image that can be printed on business cards to make tickets). On the day of the Countdown Completion, hold a raffle. Those who complete most of the aforementioned tasks, will have the most tickets in the "hat," and thus the greatest chance of winning the prize(s) of the final drawing. (If only a few people complete all 10, consider giving those participants each a reward if possible.)

Prizes should promote wellness. Suggestions include:
- gift card to a sports gear store
- gift card for a massage
- a new iPod
- iTunes gift card
- 3 or 6 month membership to a fitness facility or program
- a session with a personal trainer
- a consult with a registered dietitian
- a "Best Body Gift Basket" with all of the above!

If it is not an option to give one of the "prize" items above, consider charging $5 more than the Success Journal price for your Countdown program in order to create a fund from which to purchase prizes.

Promotion Timeline:
4-8 weeks out:
- ❏ Send out Facebook and email "teasers" to promote program awareness.
- ❏ Download and post fliers and posters from bestbodyin52.com.
- ❏ If applicable, meet with staff, personal trainers, and/or instructors to prepare for the promotion of the Countdown. Brainstorm what you could provide for staff as incentives for their participation.
- ❏ Consider hosting a Boot Camp 2-3 days a week during the program, and perhaps offer a special rate ("Buy One Get One") for the first 20 or more to sign up. Advertise the program.
- ❏ Set up registration and payment options. Go with online registration and payment if possible (include a question prompt about T-shirt size if these will be offered). Reminder: the registration form can be downloaded from bestbodyin52.com.
- ❏ Educate staff about the program details.

6 weeks out, and 4 weeks out:
❏ Media promotion (email, Facebook, website, radio, newspaper, flyers)
❏ Go through the "Support" suggestions listed above and set up those that you are planning to implement.

2 weeks out:
❏ Send out both email and Facebook reminders regarding ongoing registration, and to remind participants of the Kick-Off day and time so they can be prepared to purchase their Success Journals if they have not yet done so over the registration period (and T-shirt if desired).
❏ Order your books two weeks from the time that you need them via bestbodyin52.com if greater than 10 (or via Amazon.com if less than 10).

1 week out:
❏ Send out the email and Facebook reminders again and reach out to those that have registered.
❏ Host your Countdown Kick-Off and take final registrations.
❏ Order any final books that you may need (expect last-minute requests)

1 day before the Countdown begins:
❏ The week or day before the 52 day Countdown begins, host your Countdown Kick-Off. Set up a table and offer fruit, water bottles, and coffee in your lobby (if applicable). At the Kick-Off:
❏ take registration
❏ take payment and give participants their Success Journals
❏ get T-shirt sizes and payment for these (if applicable)
❏ do fitness assessments
❏ take weight/measurements
❏ take "before photos"

Throughout the Countdown:
❏ Encourage participants at intervals during the Countdown via email and Facebook.
❏ Send out reminders about the Best Body Tickets.

At the end of the Countdown, ideally at your Countdown Completion Celebration:
❏ Do final assessments to assess progress.
❏ Take "after photos."
❏ Hold the Best Body Ticket drawing and offer awards.
❏ Announce the date of your next Countdown, if applicable.

172

Appendix B

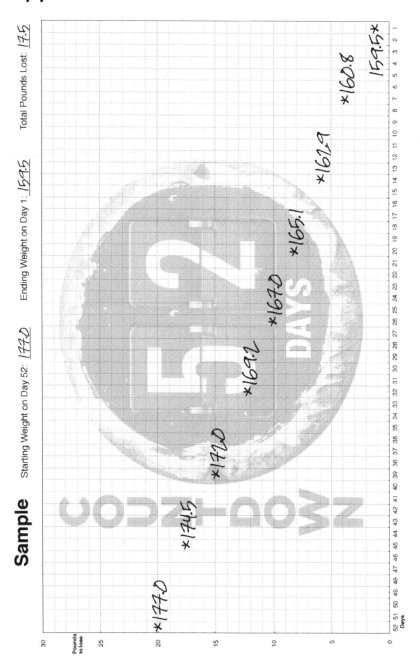

Sample   Starting Weight on Day 52: _177.0_   Ending Weight on Day 1: _159.5_   Total Pounds Lost: _17.5_

*177.0
*174.5
*172.0
*169.2
*167.0
*165.1
*161.9
*160.8
159.5*

Pounds to lose: 30, 25, 20, 15, 10, 5, 0

Days: 52 51 50 49 48 47 46 45 44 43 42 41 40 39 38 37 36 35 34 33 32 31 30 29 28 27 26 25 24 23 22 21 20 19 18 17 16 15 14 13 12 11 10 9 8 7 6 5 4 3 2 1

Appendix C

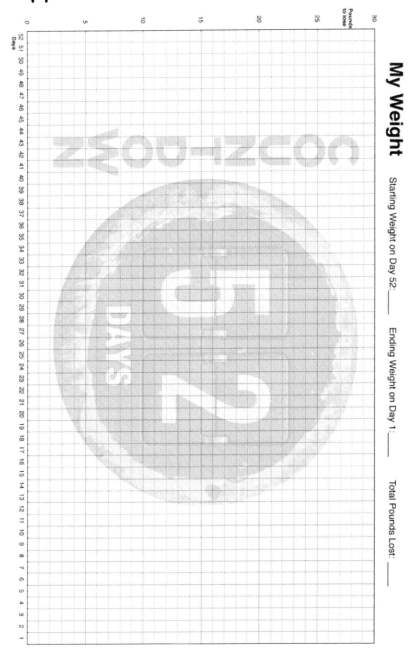

My Weight

Starting Weight on Day 52: _____

Ending Weight on Day 1: _____

Total Pounds Lost: _____

Appendix D

Exercise Tracker: Move for 52 minutes five days per week!

Days 52–39

Countdown Exercise Tracker	"Move It! Move It!"	"Don't just stand there, move!"
Goal: Check off 5 of 7 days.	Check if complete	Check if complete
Day 52		
Day 51		
Day 50		
Day 49		
Day 48		
Day 47		
Day 46		
Goal: Check off 5 of the next 7 days.		
Day 45		
Day 44		
Day 43		
Day 42		
Day 41		
Day 40		
Day 39		

Days 38–25

Countdown Exercise Tracker	"Move It! Move It!"	"Don't just stand there, move!"
Goal: Check off 5 of 7 days.	Check if complete	Check if complete
Day 38		
Day 37		
Day 36		
Day 35		
Day 34		
Day 33		
Day 32		
Goal: Check off 5 of the next 7 days.		
Day 31		
Day 30		
Day 29		
Day 28		
Day 27		
Day 26		
Day 25		

Days 24–11

Countdown Exercise Tracker	"Move It! Move It!"	"Don't just stand there, move!"
Goal: Check off 5 of 7 days.	Check if complete	Check if complete
Day 24		
Day 23		
Day 22		
Day 21		
Day 20		
Day 19		
Day 18		
Goal: Check off 5 of the next 7 days.		
Day 17		
Day 16		
Day 15		
Day 14		
Day 13		
Day 12		
Day 11		

Days 10–1

Countdown Exercise Tracker	"Move It! Move It!"	"Don't just stand there, move!"
Goal: Check off 5 of 7 days.	Check if complete	Check if complete
Day 10		
Day 9		
Day 8		
Day 7		
Day 6		
Day 5		
Day 4		
Goal: Check off 5 of the next 7 days.		
Day 3		
Day 2		
Day 1		

Appendix E

FOOD LOG DATE: _____	WHEN AND WHERE?	HUNGER BEFORE AND SATIETY AFTER
BREAKFAST		0 1 2 3 4 5 6 7 8 9 10 Starving — Content — Stuffed 0 1 2 3 4 5 6 7 8 9 10 Starving — Content — Stuffed
SNACK		0 1 2 3 4 5 6 7 8 9 10 Starving — Content — Stuffed
LUNCH		0 1 2 3 4 5 6 7 8 9 10 Starving — Content — Stuffed 0 1 2 3 4 5 6 7 8 9 10 Starving — Content — Stuffed
SNACK		0 1 2 3 4 5 6 7 8 9 10 Starving — Content — Stuffed
DINNER		0 1 2 3 4 5 6 7 8 9 10 Starving — Content — Stuffed 0 1 2 3 4 5 6 7 8 9 10 Starving — Content — Stuffed
NOTES: ☐ I REACHED MY WATER GOAL!		

176

Appendix F

My BEST BODY Shopping List (think perimeter!)

Fresh produce (did you get all colors of the rainbow?)

_____   _____
_____   _____
_____   _____
_____   _____
_____   _____

Lean protein (fish, poultry & round/loin cuts of pork/beef or tofu)

_____   _____
_____   _____
_____   _____
_____   _____
_____   _____

Whole grains, cereals and beans

_____   _____
_____   _____
_____   _____
_____   _____
_____   _____

Low sodium canned goods and dried fruits

_____   _____
_____   _____

Dairy, eggs, and frozen foods

_____   _____
_____   _____
_____   _____
_____   _____

Appendix G

MEAL PLANNING	PICTURE IT!	GROCERY NEEDS	PREPARATION TIPS
Monday's Dinner			
Tuesday's Dinner			
Wednesday's Dinner			
Thursday's Dinner			
Friday's Dinner			
Saturday's Dinner			
Sunday's Dinner			

Appendix H

From the Center for Science in the Public Interest (CSPI) Nutrition Action Healthletter - used with permission

Men & Postmenopausal Women
Centrum Men Under 50* (1)
Centrum Silver Adults 50+
Centrum Silver Men 50+
CVS Daily Multiple Tablets for Men
CVS Spectravite Adult 50+ Multivitamin
Equate Complete Multivitamin Adults 50+
Equate Complete Multivitamin Men's 50+
Equate Complete Multivitamin Women's 50+*
Equate One Daily Men's Health
Nature Made Multi for Her 50+
Nature Made Multi for Him
Nature Made Multi for Him 50+
Nature's Bounty ABC Plus Senior
Nutrilite Daily Multivitamin Multimineral*
One A Day Men's 50+ Healthy Advantage (2)
One A Day Men's Health Formula
One A Day Women's 50+ Healthy Advantage (2)
Target Up & Up Adults' Multivitamins
Walgreens A thru Z Select Multivitamin
* Contains 6 or 8 mg of iron (other multis in the list have no iron).
(1) Contains 1.3 mg of riboflavin.
(2) Contains 117 mcg of selenium

Premenopausal Women
Centrum Adults Under 50
CVS Daily Multiple Tablets for Women (1)
CVS Spectravite Ultra Women's Multivitamin (1)
Equate Complete Multivitamin Adults Under 50

Equate One Daily Women's Health (2)
Kirkland Signature Daily Multi
Nature Made Multi Complete
Nature's Bounty ABC Plus
Nature's Bounty Multi-Day Plus Minerals
Nature's Bounty Multi-Day Women's (2)
One A Day Women's
Sundown Advanced Formula SunVite
Sundown Naturals Complete Daily with Iron
Target Up & Up Multivitamin
Target Up & Up Women's Daily Multivitamin (2)
Walgreens One Daily for Women (2)
(1) Contains 25 mcg of chromium.
(2) Contains 10 mg of niacin.
If your favorite isn't on the list, it may simply not have been reviewed. You can check any label against CSPI's "What Your Multi Should Contain" list below.

What Your MULTI Should Contain

Vitamin A	No more than 5,000 IU (including any % as beta-carotene)
Vitamin C	60-1,000 mg
Vitamin D	400 IU or more
Vitamin E	20-100 IU
Vitamin K	10 mcg or more
Thiamin (B-1)	1.2 mg or more
Riboflavin (B-2)	1.7 mg or more
Niacin (B-3)	14-35 mg
Vitamin B-6	2-100 mg
Folic Acid	No more than 400 mcg
Vitamin B-12	6 mcg or more
Calcium	Don't rely on a multi
Iron	
Premenopausal women	18 mg
Everyone else	No more than 10 mg
Magnesium	50-350 mg
Zinc	No more than 30 mg
Copper	0.5-10 mg
Selenium	20-110 mcg
Chromium	35 mcg or more
Potassium	Don't rely on a multi

Appendix I: Take Tens

Minute 1: hold a plank (this will warm you up; see page 31 for instructions)
Minute 2: squats - hips level with knees before rising back up
Minute 3: 30 seconds of push-ups, 30 seconds of triceps dips
Minute 4: dance like you know you are a rock star (give it all you've got!)
Minute 5: walking lunges (if advanced, add weights)
Minute 6: jumping jacks or jump rope (beginners: quick march)
Minute 7: quick tempo squats this time (45-60 in one minute)
Minute 8: hold a plank, then move from forearms to hands, lower and repeat (do not rock through the hips while moving)
Minute 9: speed-walk or run as fast as you can
Minute 10: V-ups

Minute 1: hold a plank on your hands instead of forearms, and with your toes on the plates, draw each knee in alternately to opposite elbow while keeping hips down and naval pressed to spine, hovering over the floor
Minute 2: curtsey lunges with ball of each foot sliding the plate back, alternating right and left with fairly quick tempo (see photo)
Minute 3: 30 seconds of push-ups, 30 seconds of triceps dips
Minute 4: stand on the plates on your toes, feet together, and do a quick hip twist side to side, pushing one arm out at a time in front of you as your upper body twists opposite of your lower body
Minute 5: with the ball of each foot on a plate, do lateral shuffles (quick shuffle steps sideways across the room and back)
Minute 6: scissor shuffle - toes pointing forward, plates under feet in tandem foot position, switching feet in a scissoring motion; arms like you're running
Minute 7: stand as wide as you can on

the plates, toes out and hips low: 1) bring feet together with a quick hop, standing taller as you draw feet in; 2) slide out with a little scoot and repeat (as you get more comfortable with this, you can do it more briskly)
Minute 8: single-leg dead lift (weighted if desired), 10 R, 10 L and repeat (see above)
Minute 9: "mountain climbers" with balls of feet on discs/plates (see photo, left)
Minute 10: basic crunches

Minute 1: punching bag arms (increasing speed as you warm up), while holding a wide, low squat (toes out) - 30 sec R, 30 sec L
Minute 2: 30-second plank*; (beginners, continue with plank hold; advanced, do squat thrusts/burpees for the second 30 seconds)
Minute 3: sprinter pulls* (aka "screamers") - 10 R, 10 L; repeat
Minute 4: side plank with straight leg* (bent lower leg for beginners) - 30 sec R, 30 sec L
Minute 5: lunge forward R (knee over ankle), step feet together, and lunge back L, step feet together - 30 seconds, then switch lead leg for 30 seconds
Minute 6: 30 sec pushups, 30 sec triceps dips
Minute 7: fast feet (sprint in place) - 30 seconds; wall squat - hold for 30 seconds (back flat against the wall, legs in front as if seated in an imaginary chair)
Minute 8: explosive jump up on a step or stair, then step down, repeat
Minute 9: hold your balance while doing a side kick with 1 leg with a quick toe tap down before lifting for another side kick - 30 sec R side, 30 sec L; allow yourself an extra moment of slow moving to cool down before finishing with abs in Minute 10
Minute 10: supine bicycle crunches*

180

Appendix J

Serving Sizes — hint: 1 grain or starch = 15 g carb; limit or avoid those along the bottom

Meats	Vegetables	Grain/Starch	Fruit	Dairy	Fat
Fish (not fried) Salmon, trout, herring, flounder, mackerel, tuna, and others	1 cup raw vegetables ½ cup cooked or finely chopped vegetables	1/3 cup cooked rice 1/2 cup cooked pasta, oats, quinoa, bulgur, or barley	1 tennis ball-sized fruit such as an apple, peach, etc. ½ banana	1 cup skim or 1% milk 1 cup yogurt, regular or Greek yogurt	2 tbsp. avocado (1/5) 8 olives 4–10 nuts 1 ½ tsp nut butter 1 tbsp. sunflower, pumpkin, or flax seeds
Poultry: White meat, no skin	starchy vegetables and beans are counted with grains because of their starchy quality	½ cup grits 6 saltine-size crackers or 2 crisp-breads	¾ cup any berries 1 cup any melon cubes	1.5 oz fat-free or reduced-fat cheese Mozzarella, ricotta, and feta are naturally lower in fat	1 tsp. oil 1 tbsp. Promise or Smart Balance spread
Beef and Pork: Loin and round cuts are typically lean		1 slice whole-grain bread (1 ounce)	½ cup applesauce, unsweetened		1 tbsp. salad dressing (2 if tbsp. light) dressing
lean lunch meat (limit nitrates) 1 egg = 1 oz. meat		½ whole wheat pita or English muffin ¾ cup whole-grain cereal 1/2 cup of corn, peas, potatoes, sweet potatoes, or beans	2 tbsp. dried fruits 4 ounces 100% juice	¼ cup low-fat cottage cheese	2 tsp. mayo 1 tsp. coconut oil 1 tsp. butter 1 tbsp. cream cheese
Avoid: Bologna, bacon, sausage, salami, hot dogs, and limit highly processed deli meats		Limit: White or refined grain products, biscuits, cornbread, granola, fried potatoes, waffles, cookies, and cakes	Limit: Juice, fruit drinks	Limit: Whole milk, full-fat cheeses and yogurts, ice cream, cream soups	Limit or Avoid: Butter, cream soups, stick margarine, bacon, fatback, gravy, cream, shortening, full-fat dressings, and hydrogenated oils (trans fat) in packaged products

Appendix K
"Fueling" for Your Best Body

Sample Day

This sample day is about 1600 calories. See a registered dietitian to customize your calorie level, as 1600 calories is not appropriate for all.

Breakfast: 7 AM
black coffee (sweeten with Stevia or Splenda if needed)
1 cup of fat free or 1% milk (to drink, or mix in oatmeal or coffee)
1/2 cup cooked old fashioned oatmeal with 1/2 teaspoon brown sugar added
1 slice of whole wheat toast with 1 1/2 teaspoons peanut butter
1 orange, whole (or choose another fruit to mix into oatmeal)
water

10:30 AM: 1 apple and sparkling water with no additives

Lunch: 12:00 PM
3 ounces of tuna with 1 1/2 teaspoons light mayo, add 1/2 cup of finely chopped raw spinach and stir it in (try the food processor to chop)
4 Ryvita Sesame Rye crisp-bread crackers
1 cup Refreshing Rainbow Salad (see Day 51 for recipe)
water

"Strong Snack:" 3:30 PM
8 ounces (1 cup) unsweetened Greek yogurt with 3/4 cup mixed blueberries and strawberries and 1/2 teaspoon honey if needed
6 almonds
hot or chilled peppermint tea, unsweetened

Dinner: 6:30 PM
Perfectly Filling Lettuce Wraps (see Day 40 for recipe)
3 1/2 ounce chicken breast, marinated in The Perfect Dressing (see Day 47 for recipe)
unsweetened tea with lemon

FAQ and Topic Search

About the Author

Sohailla Digsby, RD, LD

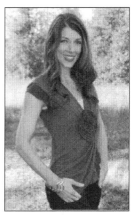 Sohailla Digsby is a registered dietitian and fitness instructor. She started teaching aerobics when she was studying nutrition at the University of Georgia in the 1990s. Whether she's writing, presenting, teaching Zumba, developing wellness programs, leading boot camp, or consulting nutrition clients, Sohailla loves to motivate people to be their best physically. She is passionate about keeping her message balanced and realistic, knowing that after the hype of the fads fade, people simply need practical steps to build a foundation that will last.

During a typical day you might find her in heels making a presentation, later in sneakers jogging alongside her kids as they bike in the neighborhood while a crock-pot dinner simmers, and then around the dinner table in her slippers with her family. She is multi-tasking through every 52 days, just like you, and wants you to be encouraged that once the Best-Body foundation is built for a healthy lifestyle, it becomes a way of life that doesn't take extremes to maintain. Sohailla prioritizes making health and fitness fun, practical, and memorable so all of you will be compelled to do the same for the long-haul!

To find out when the accompanying publications to the Success Journal are being released, and more about why Sohailla chose exactly 52 days for the Countdown, stay in touch through bestbodyin52.com.

To my wonderful family, friends, clients, and interns whose many nutrition and fitness questions spurred me to put the answers all in one place.

A heartfelt thanks to God for the inspiration for this book and the drive to see it through. I am beyond grateful to my precious husband and loved ones for their helping hands that allowed me to complete this book during a busy season of life.

Made in the USA
Charleston, SC
27 August 2014